THE LAW OF NATURAL HEALING

SUGGESTION

First Edition 1906
Charles L Gilson

New Edition 2019
Edited by Tarl Warwick

COPYRIGHT AND DISCLAIMER

FOREWORD

The author of this text, Charles Gilson, is mostly known for strictly fictional works, but "The Law of Natural Healing" is an extremely interesting book- specifically, it proposes that suggestion is of help for virtually all then-common diseases and symptoms within the lexicon of medicine.

The book is definitively a product of its era; Tuberculosis is referred to as the "American Disease" (it has been virtually eliminated in the USA in the modern era) and no mention of iodine deficiency is made in regards to goiter- however, in the strictly theoretical sense, suggestion is potentially useful in some of the contexts listed here; especially regarding addiction to tobacco and alcohol- it is still resorted to (with various degrees of success) by people seeking treatment for the same, even if auto-suggestion has "mostly" fallen from grace in mainstream medicine. Self-hypnosis is also spoken of here. Such a practice is less common than the use of hypnosis, these days, for amusement.

It ought to be duly noted that some of the diseases here are potentially life threatening and any indication of their presence should result in the consultation of medical professionals.

This edition of "The Law of Natural Healing" has been carefully edited for format and content. Care has been taken to retain all original intent and meaning.

THE LAW OF NATURAL HEALING

TO MY MOTHER

who knew my aims and my hopes;
who believed in me and my work,
this book is reverently dedicated.

THE LAW OF NATURAL HEALING

PREFACE

In preparing this series of lessons upon the art of Natural Healing, I have entertained no intention of entering into abstruse discussions of the laws of mental or psychic phenomena. These laws have long since been adequately formulated and discussed by such eminent writers as Dr. Hudson and others, and I have no need to speak of them except to illustrate and make clear the harmony that exists between my own work and the great principles of natural law. I wish most emphatically to state in the beginning that I claim nothing outside the rigid and fast-fixed boundaries of definitely understood psychic phenomena. There is nothing supernatural, nothing transcending Nature's immutable law, in what I have done. I have but applied laws and reaped the beneficent results of abiding within the law- no act of mine has for an instant controverted or opposed the great, simple, unchangeable statutes that Mother Nature has written in indelible characters for the guidance of her universal creation.

Any man who claims powers outside these laws, or any man who claims ability to set them at naught with impunity, may be set down unhesitatingly as ignorant or an impostor. Nor have I any intention of entering into any campaign against any now-established theory or system of treating or healing the sick. I believe that all systems of healing have some substance of truth and do a certain amount of good, else they could not exist. The world has seen innumerable systems of theology, philosophy and sociology, each with its partisans convinced of its complete infallibility. Some of these systems have been so choked with error and absurdity that today we merely laugh at their vagaries, yet unbiased inspection of their principles will almost invariably reveal a kernel of unalloyed truth at the bottom. The wildest theory man ever evolved probably had in its inception some minute revelation of immutable law, perhaps disclosed only as is caught a glimpse of some far-away shining mountain peak, never before seen, though dimly and intuitively believed to exist, but instantly swallowed up again in impenetrable cloud and mystery. So it is only the narrow and the self-sufficient man who denies that his neighbor has even glimpsed the summit, when he himself claims to be gazing from another angle at its fully unveiled effulgence. Truth is always potent, and a very little infusion of it "leaveneth a whole lump" of error and misconception. It is only to be regretted that so many modem systems of healing are hampered and choked into comparative uselessness by a cumbersome mechanism of tradition, dogma, etiquette, prejudice and narrowness.

I claim only to have cast off these irksome bonds which hamper so many conscientious workers in the great field of alleviating human suffering and pain, and by so doing to have used the truth and discarded the dross. I have ever aimed to get back close to Nature- to use her methods and to give unquestioning obedience to her laws. That is why my system of Natural Healing, as I have always preferred to call it, has proved itself so efficacious as it has. It is Nature's own way and therefore is not a man-made system at all, not the creation of my brain or any other man's, but simply a right system of doing Nature's own bidding. I have formed and coordinated the plan of healing and made it available, but I could no more have created it than I could create the universe. This, then, is my reason for offering this book to the public- that all may freely know of the results I have obtained in a long practice full of seemingly miraculous curative successes; secondly, how I have obtained them; and lastly, that all who will, may learn to attain like results themselves.

I claim that, with the assistance of this volume, any person of suitable physical, mental and moral make-up, may heal the sick and banish pain without medicine or surgery, as easily and efficaciously as I have been doing it daily for years.

CHAPTER I

MOST POWERFUL SERVANT - HELP IS FROM WITHIN -
THE SUBJECTIVE MIND - KNOWLEDGE OF ITS
FUNCTIONS PREREQUISITE TO HEALTH CONCEPTIONS
OF FAITH - "KNOW THYSELF, THEN HELP THYSELF AND
OTHERS"

This book is calculated to teach the principles of Natural Healing. I do not anticipate that every person who reads it will be able to cure disease. Any person who reads it and assimilates its contents can do so if he choose, but very many will not. That is always to be assumed with reference to any subject of instruction. Very many students annually matriculate at the various institutions of learning throughout the world, and very few actually become experts in the subjects they elect to study. One has to look but a short distance in his own vicinity to find some one who has acquired all the book knowledge of a profession, or all the theory of a science and yet is neither able to apply his knowledge practically nor to teach it to others. Such knowledge is not, however, acquired in vain, for though the person may not benefit himself or others in a material way by what he has learned, still the very fact of his knowing is helpful to him. Particularly is the above true with reference to knowledge acquired along the lines of mental phenomena. A right understanding of the principles which govern mental therapeutics cannot fail to be of benefit to any student, no matter whether he studies to know and apply his knowledge or merely to know alone. So I claim that a careful perusal of this volume will be helpful to any person of intelligence, whether he aims simply to help himself or if he has the higher ambition of helping his fellow men.

The first and most essential prerequisite in the study of this book is that the student should know whence comes the power with which he deals and by means of which he works. Without such knowledge, the student is manifestly entirely at sea and all his efforts entirely futile. So it may fairly be said that the remainder of this chapter contains the absolute first essential to an understanding of the subject, and should be carefully assimilated by the reader regardless of the object with which he approaches the study. There is just one thing always to be kept rigidly in view, namely, "The mind is the source of all curative power." An understanding of this dictum is the key to the art of Natural Healing.

The human mind is, without any question, a dual entity. It consists of two distinct elements each essential to the other and to life. Each has separate and well-understood functions, and each may act entirely independently of the other. These two halves of the mental entity are called: I. The Objective, or conscious mind; II. The Subjective, or subconscious mind.

The Objective mind is that portion of the human mentality, through which we are cognizant of exterior facts. It is that portion of the mind which perceives, through the medium of the five senses, the conditions and events which go on outside ourselves, and by which we are conscious of their effect upon ourselves. It is also the reasoning mind and possesses- the power of logic or the power of reasoning from cause to effect and vice-versa. The Subjective mind, on the contrary, is the portion of the mind which controls all the sensations, emotions and functions of the body. It cannot reason, but it is gifted with infallible memory. It is the indelible record upon which is written down every experience of life. It is the absolute master of every atom of the physical being of man. It is the spirit.

All that man needs to acquire perfect mastery over himself is the power to make the Subjective mind his servant. Of course this sounds to the uninitiated an impossible requirement, but in reality it is the simplest. All we need to realize is that The power which regenerates, the power which makes us whole, is within ourselves. GOD IS WITHIN us, not far away in some inaccessible Heaven where only the elect may hope to climb, but His Spirit is within every one of his living creatures. We have only to assert our real selves to become Godlike. How strange a thing it is that so marvelous a truth should have been lost and ever sought after, now and again half regrasped only to be lost again, throughout the ages! Ever has man sought far afield for the power to overcome disease and death, while all the time it lay within the confines of his own being. It is like the allegory of Hawthorne in which the peasant boy waits patiently his lifetime for the fabled poet to appear, only to find at last that he himself is the chosen one.

Within every man there is the absolute power of controlling his own destiny, within reasonable limits, and this applies first of all to the control of his physical existence. It is self-evident that if the Subjective mind controls the functions of the body, it is simply necessary to control the Subjective mind in order to dictate the perfect working of the body. The Subjective mind is to be likened to the careful housekeeper, who, when her activities are properly directed, so orders the domicile that every factor of life moves smoothly within it, and makes it an ideal dwelling-place. The Subjective mind, when properly directed through the medium of the will, coordinates the functions and keeps the human temple a dwelling-place fit for its divine tenant, the Soul. In no way is the beautiful simplicity of divine law more notably shown than in the relation of mankind to the power which he possesses within himself. The Subjective mind is without question the spark of divine life in man. Yet it is entirely within his power of control. Subtle and mysterious as the Subjective entity is, it is ever amenable to Objective suggestion. Reason, which is, contrary to the often repeated dictum of the poet, not the divine attribute of man at all, but merely a human one, is capable of directing the Subjective mind through the medium of the will. The Objective mind, which depends for its acts upon reason, which vanishes with consciousness and which dies with the physical body, can compel the undying spirit to do its behests.

In a single word. The Subjective mind is always amenable to Objective suggestion. The will is the connecting link between the two entities. The Subjective mind, being incapable of reason or logic, acts upon every thought of the Objective mind, that is, upon every suggestion given it. "As a man thinketh, so is he," is absolutely a statement of fact. Now right at this point some students will say, "Why, this is simply 'Faith cure,' and as I could never have faith enough to cure either myself or others, this method will be of no advantage to me." There could be no greater mistake than that.

Faith is essential to the cure of disease, no matter by what means it is attempted. Nothing in the world can be done without Faith. The man who does not believe in himself can never do anything or be anything worth while. It makes no difference what the nature of the belief is, a belief of some sort is essential to success in the most trivial thing as well as in the greatest activity of life. We could not even breathe if we did not have faith that our lungs would fill themselves so many times a minute without effort on our own part. A man carries a potato in his pocket to cure rheumatism, but it is his faith and not the potato that effects the cure. The great trouble with those who decry so-called Faith cure is that they know only Objective faith. They wholly disregard Subjective faith, and it is Subjective faith that cures disease. Objective faith directs the curative power, but Subjective faith is that power.

Here again is illustrated Nature's wonderful providence of an infallible remedy for man's ills. Faith is an essential requisite, but man cannot always command reason to have it-that is, he cannot always have Objective faith. So then, Nature provides the possibility of Subjective faith, independent of anything but mechanical means. In other words, repetition will create Subjective faith regardless of reason. It is only necessary to repeat a suggestion, either for good or evil, to the Subjective mind and it will act upon it, no matter whether the conscious mind believes it or not. The repetition of a suggestion is an infallible creator of Subjective belief and consequent action, for the Subjective mind acts upon every suggestion which it accepts-that is, in which it gains faith.

If Objective faith were the basis of "Faith-cure" so-called, "Faith-cure," mental healing and Natural Healing would all alike be fallacious. It is a deeper, more spiritual quality that we mean when we say that faith is essential to healing. It is not the faith of logic or of reason, but the faith of the spirit which cures.

When the Savior said "The Kingdom of God is within you," he referred to just this fact, that the power which makes man Godlike rests within himself, and is his by divine birthright, the power to surmount the weakness of the flesh by the inherent attributes of the spirit. So when He further said, "Except ye become as a little child, ye cannot enter into the Kingdom of Heaven," He emphasized the need for recognizing Subjective faith and its basic Naturalness, rather than for depending upon the evanescent attributes of the Objective entity. The one is Natural and infallible because it is spiritual and immortal, the other is complicated with constant possibility of error because it is physical and mortal. Briefly to sum up, then, the student must first gain a true conception of the fact that he has within himself a power which needs only to be applied in order to overcome all physical obstacles. The limits of accomplishment are determined only by the student's own personal ability to grasp the theory of Subjective force and to develop and apply the forces of his own being.

Understand first that you have within yourself the key to

power. Determine that you will develop that power. Believe in yourself. Know that you can do and be what you will, within natural limits. Remember that you have the most wonderful force in the universe within yourself, and that you need only to know how to apply it to become master of disease. Suggestion is the lever which controls the current of vital force.

Practice is the only thing needful after theory has been acquired. Cultivate faith in yourself and you will instill it into others. Learn to distinguish between the Objective faith which reason teaches that you may well have in the constant operation of Natural laws, and the Subjective faith which you will need to cultivate by means of repeated suggestion in the subconscious mentality of your patients. "Know thyself, then help thyself and others."

With each succeeding day of practice in controlling the Subjective mind by means of suggestion, you will find new power and strength becoming your own. There is no limit to your possibilities if you will determine to he yourself. In succeeding chapters I will endeavor to describe practical applications of the grand law of suggestion, but first let the student Now that in his own breast is the secret of all power.

THE LAW OF NATURAL HEALING

CHAPTER II

PREPARATION FOR TREATMENT – OPERATOR SELF
TRAINED – CONFIDENCE IN SELF AND CONFIDENCE OF
PATIENT – METHODS OF IMPLANTING FAITH –
METHODS OF SUGGESTION – EXPECTANT ATTENTION

It is of course to be assumed that previous to attempting the healing of the sick, the student will have thoroughly mastered the theory of suggestion as the foundation of all curative power. He will have trained his own Subjective entity to control the functions of his own body, and he will by long practice have accustomed himself to think always in terms of Natural Science- that is, he will have reached a state of mind in which the Subjective and Objective minds act together in accordance with the principles heretofore laid down. He will always know that in himself is the one agency which can overcome material obstacles, and he will have gone beyond the stage where doubt is possible because he knows there can be no doubt of the Subjective power.

Assuming then, that the student is ready to apply his knowledge to relieving others, he should first of all consider the element of confidence. The operator should first have complete confidence in himself, or rather, in the power that is within himself, and secondly, he should aim to secure the confidence of the patient. Too much stress cannot be placed upon the importance of making an initial good impression. Everybody knows how essential a good first impression is in any affair of life. First impressions may not always be reliable, but they are generally the most influential. I have already discussed the need of faith in order to heal. Securing Objective faith is the easiest method of assuring Subjective faith. If you believe in yourself, and show it by an air of quiet strength and confidence, the patient also will believe in you, and the moment he does so, you can be sure you can cure him. The reason for that is simply that the Objective faith which he conceives in you, engendered by your strength of personality, induces in him Subjective faith, or in other words, you are yourself a most potent suggestion to the patient.

You will never induce faith in a patient by telling him that he must have it in order to be cured. Such a procedure would be an adverse suggestion that you might never afterwards be able to overcome. But if a patient is manifestly skeptical, it is your business to overcome that prejudice as your own best judgment may dictate for each individual case. Of course it is in this respect that each student's own personal tact and ability will determine his success. Some patients may be argued with, others can be won to belief in you by a gradual process of securing their friendship and others must be shown cases parallel to their own, where the result has been beneficial either through your own efforts or those of other mental practitioners. Each patient must be handled carefully and the student's own tact and "skill in handling people," as the expression is, will determine the measure of his success. Suggestion is always the basis of Natural Healing, but suggestion takes various forms, and skill and judgment must x always be used in selecting the right form to apply to each individual case.

Various methods will have to be used with different patients. With some it is best to place the hands upon the affected parts, with others simply the glance accompanied by appropriate suggestions is all that is required, while with others various mechanical expedients may be employed as suggested by the experience and ingenuity of the operator. All that is necessary is to obtain the attention and hence the cooperation of the patient. It is always to be remembered that all mechanical expedients are but forms of suggestion and have in themselves no virtue whatever except as they assist in attracting the Objective attention and thus influencing the Subjective entity.

THE LAW OF NATURAL HEALING

It is well known that it is only necessary to fix the attention firmly upon a portion of the body in order to affect its physical condition. Thus it is perfectly possible to slow down or to accelerate the pulse by fixing the attention upon the heart. Many nervous persons can so affect their heart action as to produce fainting merely because they expect they are going to faint.

The phenomena of expectant attention are many and varied. There are scores of well-authenticated instances in which constant dwelling upon the fear of disease has produced it in due time. This is especially true with reference to cancer, hydrophobia, tuberculosis and other diseases of more or less obscure nature which from their malignancy are particularly objects of popular apprehension. A very recent case reported in the newspapers occurred in Chicago. A young man named Johnson, about six months previously to his death, had owned a small dog which was bitten by another animal and died of rabies. Johnson was never bitten by the animal nor was he ever really in danger from the affair, but he constantly brooded upon it and finally began to exhibit all the symptoms of hydrophobia.

He finally died in the utmost agony, though it was perfectly well known that he could never by any possibility have contracted the malady from any exterior source. This was a typical case of expectant attention resulting in actual simulation of disease. His constant Objective fear reacted upon the Subjective mind until the actual condition of disease was produced.

Every New England born person can, if he lived in the country, look back to his childhood and remember being told that poison-ivy would injure only those who feared it. There is excellent reason for believing that this is the fact, for many cases have been observed in which people touched the plant without knowing what it was until some time afterward, and received no harm whatever, while in other cases the first symptoms of poisoning followed shortly after learning the nature of the plant. In exactly the same way, many an instance has been recorded of people being practically frightened to death by the bite of some reptile which they thought venomous but which really was not so. In some instances the discovery of the innocuous nature of the creature was made in time to cause a laughably quick recovery from apparently imminent dissolution.

So when the attention of a patient is brought to a portion of the body by repeated suggestion, it is possible to affect the status of that member in a great many ways. If there is inflammation, the attention is directed to the part, and the suggestion given is that the blood is receding from it, that there is a marked decrease in the tension there, that a feeling of coolness and relief exists and that the tissues are losing the superabundance of blood supply. On the other hand, where there is restriction of the circulation, such as occurs in paralysis of some kinds, the reverse process is employed, and in response the circulation will be quickened, the tissues filled with fresh blood and thus renovated.

CHAPTER III

General Methods

TONING UP GENERAL SYSTEM - IMPORTANCE OF
SOLAR PLEXUS IN SUGGESTIVE TREATMENT - HOW TO
STIMULATE CIRCULATION AND DIGESTION - EFFECTS
OF GENERAL TREATMENT – WHEN NAUSEA IS AN
ENCOURAGING SYMPTOM - SUGGESTIVE USE OF
WATER - MAGNETIZED WATER - ADAPTING
TREATMENT TO INDIVIDUAL CASES - VITAL
NECESSITY OF CO-OPERATION BETWEEN PATIENT AND
HEALER

Every good method to use in treating cases of a general
nature wherein it is desired to tone up the whole system and thus
aid nature to restore the normal tone to the whole body, is as
follows. It is well to seat the patient in a comfortable chair or
allow him to recline with the head and shoulders slightly raised.
You may then spend a few minutes in talking quietly with him,
explaining that the treatment you are about to give him will
cause his circulation to become better, the nervous energy to be
increased and the general system toned up. Here again the
operator must use his skill and judgment in determining what to
tell the patient. The operator must use his personal knowledge of
his patient and adapt his explanations to the patient's normal
intellect and ability to understand, as well as to his present
condition. Sometimes patients are in such a weakened or
debilitated condition that too much talking of any kind is hurtful
to them. Tact alone can determine the course for each individual
case.

When you have secured the attention of the patient, look
fixedly at him, meeting his eyes and holding his attention
without staring at him. Place the right hand upon the pit of the

patient's stomach, calling his attention to the fact that it is the location of the solar plexus, which is considered to be the seat of vital energy. It is the most important nerve plexus in the body and it is believed that it governs the sympathetic nerve system and the organic functions almost entirely.

Tell the patient that this is the case, and that you are imparting to the plexus a stimulation which will cause it to resume activity. It will thus increase the secretions of the stomach, the liver and the intestines, the bile will flow more freely, the processes of digestion will go on normally and the colon will be lubricated so that movements will be normal. The kidneys will also be stimulated to activity. All the time that these explanations are being given in a quiet, firm tone, in language suited to the patient's condition and understanding, the operator's hand should be slowly describing a rectangular path upon the abdomen, following the course of the colon. A vibratory motion may also be given gently over the seat of the solar plexus, at the moment when it is stated that the object is to stimulate that organ in its functions. This treatment, you may proceed to say, will correct all digestive troubles and will thus give Nature a chance to make new blood and tissue to replace the ravages of disease. In cases of nervous debility, this treatment may be supplemented by seating the patient in such manner that his spine can be easily reached, and then placing the left hand upon the back of the patient's neck at the base of the brain, while the right hand is used to make passes slowly along the spinal column. In all cases the treatment should conclude with appropriate suggestions to the effect that improvement will be noticed immediately in the digestive and other functions, and that pain, if any exist, will disappear.

The treatments described above are of course general ones and should be in addition to special treatments for local disorders. The seat of pain, if any exist, must always be treated locally, in addition to general treatment, and if pain is severe, attention will of course be given to relieving it before anything else is done. It has often happened in my practice that patients treated in the general manner I have described will complain that within a few hours after the first treatment, they experienced unusual discomfort and in some cases violent nausea. This I believe to be caused by the stimulation of the nervous system and the stirring up of the abdominal organs together with the effort thus made to throw off stagnant secretions and impurities. I have always found that patients who experienced this phenomenon were the quickest and most completely cured, and I always make use of this fact as a potent suggestion to aid their further progress. Naturally some patients are much discouraged by this sudden turn for the worse, as it seems to them to be, and if the operator has reason to believe his patient may be one liable to this experience, he may warn the patient in advance not to feel worried, as it is exactly what is desired and looked for. It is a fact that I have found it a most favorable and desirable indication of recovery. I have noted the same phenomenon in cases of neuralgia and sciatica, where a tremendous paroxysm of pain followed the first treatment within a few hours- and then never reappeared in any form, the patient being completely cured.

I have found the use of water very valuable in many ways. Of course liberal drinking of pure water is a hygienic precaution that a great many people neglect, and the student will often find cases where all the patient requires is to drink a needful supply of pure water daily. Many a $100 fee has been paid to specialists on digestive diseases for the simple advice, "drink water."

But in addition to this, water may be made to serve real curative as well as preventive purposes. In cases of dyspepsia, constipation and allied troubles, the operator may draw a glass of water and call the patient's attention to it, not necessarily in words, but by giving the impression of much importance attaching to it. Set the glass upon the palm of the left hand, and place the right over its top, imparting a vibrating motion to the hands in such manner that the patient sees you are doing so. If thought proper to do so, the suggestion may be given that you are imparting magnetic or nervous energy to the water for the patient's benefit. In some cases it may be well to breathe slightly upon the surface of the water, but in any event, the object is to give the suggestion of its efficacy to the patient. Then have the patient drink the water, giving the needful suggestions as to the effect it will have. I have seen constipation of long standing relieved by one such treatment and cured in a few more. In exactly the same way, too great activity of the bowels is relieved, the suggestions only being varied to meet the case.

It will depend, as I have said, only upon the personality of the operator, as to how potent he succeeds in making his suggestions. I have had patients declare the water I prepared for them to be as "prickly" in taste as vichy, while others could feel a thrill like that imparted by a galvanic battery, whenever I laid my hands upon them. These were by no means among the least intelligent of my patients, but they were among those most easily benefited. They were those in whom Objective faith was easily implanted and they did not, like others, have to be given a long course of repeated suggestions in order to create Subjective faith.

The operator ought always to remember that each individual patient may be expected to exhibit new peculiarities of physical and temperamental make-up. No two patients will react in exactly the same manner and what may benefit one, may have no effect upon another. Neither is it possible to generalize as to the outcome of cases. I have seen in my practice two cases of the same disease which seemed almost identical as to nature and progress of the malady, age and general condition of the patient, etc., yet one might be cured in a single treatment and the other not till after several weeks of constant attendance. Why this should be so cannot be explained except upon the ground of difference in temperament, and obscure subjective phenomena.

THE LAW OF NATURAL HEALING

So it is never well to make prophecies as to the length of time necessary to cure a patient nor to attempt to generalize from special cases. It must not be supposed that failures do not occasionally occur in Natural Healing as well as in all other human endeavors. No matter how infallible a law or a theory may be, human application of it is always fraught with the danger of failure. One of the greatest obstacles to unfailing success is the difficulty of securing positive cooperation between operator and patient. The patient must cooperate or he cannot hope to be cured.

One of the most vital differences between Natural Healing and so-called "faith cure" is that the latter implies a miraculous cure of disease in answer to prayer or to objective faith. It implies that a petition to God can induce Him to change His immutable laws in a given instance. It implies that God, instead of being unchangeable as He has Himself declared He is, is really vacillating and capable of being induced to change the whole course of universal law in answer to the petition of an individual. In other words, if "faith cure" were a tenable proposition, every manifestation of it would be a miracle and a revocation of Natural law.

So then, it often happens that a patient is found who looks for an immediate and magical recovery. He wants to be rid of a condition in a minute that it took months of abuse of Nature to produce. He shuts his mind to the operator's explanations and suggestions and waits for some magical hocus-pocus to restore him to youth and strength instantly. Needless to say, such an event does not occur. Then he gives up the treatment in a fine scorn and disgust of such "'quackery." Natural Healing requires more than the swallowing of a drug or a potion. It requires knowledge. Some patients unconsciously oppose their whole wills to the operator's efforts. They subconsciously determine that nothing whatever shall be allowed to controvert their own particular set habits of thought. They may assure the operator that they place themselves unreservedly in his hands, yet, perhaps unconsciously to themselves, they are set in the purpose to let nothing combat their own creeds, dogmas and habitual beliefs. Such patients also shut their minds against helpful suggestion and knowledge and cannot be helped so long as they maintain this attitude. In all such cases, to use the language of Natural Healing, they defeat your suggestions by stronger adverse auto-suggestions.

But if a patient will open his mind to knowledge, and faithfully comply with mental laws, good effects are impossible to avoid for they follow in natural sequence. Oftentimes there are subjective causes which will aid or retard progress, but these can only be dealt with individually. The mind tainted with selfishness, covetousness, avarice, sensuality or jealousy shuts itself to help. The relations between operator and patient should be made as intimate as can be accomplished, without the loss of dignity on the part of the operator. Too much familiarity breeds contempt is as true in regard to the relation of healer and patient as it is in any other application to earthly affairs.

The operator ought to strive to gain the respect, esteem and confidence of his subject, and the only way in which this can be done is by being worthy of such respect and esteem. You can never do a patient good unless you approach his case with a sincere desire to benefit him, not for the effect it will have upon your own fame or purse, but because of the good you are going to do him. If you approach each case in your practice with an earnest effort and intent to help the patient for his own sake, you will gain success, but otherwise you will not do so to any such extent as will the man whose heart is filled with pity and love for suffering humanity. Love for one's fellow men is absolutely necessary in order to get the best results by Natural Healing methods. In no other way than by a sincere and unfeigned sympathy with suffering fellow mortals can you really secure their confidence. The evidences and sentiments of compassion cannot be simulated without ultimate detection. You may not be conscious that your affectation of sympathy is detected, but the results will show themselves unfailingly in your practice.

The more a healer gives out to his patients, the more good he himself receives. It is the true interpretation of the saying that "virtue is its own reward." The more good you give out, the more good you yourself receive. It is the true law of compensation, and the healer whose heart overflows with sympathy and love for the suffering will find his good thoughts and deeds returned to himself in ten-fold measure.

CHAPTER IV

Auto-Suggestion

COOPERATION SECURED BY SELF-GIVEN
SUGGESTIONS – MAKING TREATMENT CONTINUOUS -
HOW SUBJECTIVE FAITH IS BEST SECURED - WHEN
AUTO-SUGGESTIONS SUCCEED BEST - SIMPLE
SUGGESTIONS MOST EFFECTIVE - METHODS OF
ADMINISTERING SELF-HELP

Suggestion is the basis of Natural Healing. It makes no difference what the suggestion is nor from whence it emanates, it will control the subjective mind, if not controverted by stronger suggestion. So then the student must in the beginning furnish suggestions to himself before he begins to treat others. It is by the suggestions he gives himself that his own subjective mind is controlled, so it is obvious that he can instruct his patients how to help themselves in the same manner. The need for cooperation between patient and operator has been emphasized before. There is no way in which such cooperation can be better secured than by teaching the patient the principles of auto-suggestion. If the patient practices autosuggestion systematically under right guidance by the operator, he makes his treatment a continuous one and the efforts of the operator are supplemented in a most effective manner.

It has been stated that subjective faith is generated by repetition of suggestions, hence the value of auto-suggestion cannot be overestimated in this connection. The most difficult cases of objective opposition to cure by Natural means, can be overcome by auto-suggestion if persisted in. The operator, having secured the attention of the patient and gotten him interested in the treatment, may tell him that he can aid in his own recovery by a few minutes' treatment daily. The operator can then explain the necessity for governing the subjective mind by appropriate suggestions and may dictate some suggestions to the patient to be repeated at certain intervals during the day. Most patients will grasp the idea immediately and proceed to arrange suitable suggestions for themselves, and by applying them will hasten their recoveries by many days. It is obvious that the patient who depends solely upon the operator for the good he is to receive will not progress as rapidly as the one who trains his own subjective mind to a continuous, though subconscious, process of self-help.

Auto-suggestions may be given helpfully at all times, though they succeed best when given regularly and systematically. Suggestions are to the mind what exercise is to the body, in this respect. It has, however, been shown by repeated experiments that suggestions are most potent when given just before the patient falls asleep. The objective mind vanishes, to all intents and purposes, when unconsciousness comes. So far as the objective mind is concerned, sleep is as conclusive as death. But the subjective mind is even more active during sleep than during waking hours. Suggestions given just before sleep is induced seem to repeat themselves mechanically during sleep and thus acquire their very fullest effect. The subjective mind is left unhampered during sleep by the possibly adverse suggestions of the objective mind, and it also has the greatest effect at that time upon the functions, especially those of circulation and digestion. If it is strongly suggested just before going to sleep that these functions are to be greatly strengthened during the ensuing sleeping hours, it will be found almost infallibly that just that effect will be obtained.

So if the patient gives himself proper auto-suggestions each night when composing himself to rest, he will do as much for himself as the operator can do for him. Some patients cannot use auto-suggestion as successfully as others, of course, but here again temperamental differences and limitations come in and must be recognized as factors in the progress of the cure. With some patients it might not be well to try to use auto-suggestion for the reason that if they were skeptical in the first place, they might misunderstand your explanations and become more skeptical. So many people have become accustomed to swallowing some sort of drug when sick and relying entirely upon that to effect a cure, that they are suspicious and distrustful the moment you suggest any self-help. The nature of auto-suggestions to be given in cases where it seems advisable to use this method must depend upon the individual and upon the disease. Patients suffering much pain will be less likely to make good use of auto-suggestions than others, though in cases where they are fully convinced of the efficacy of the method, self-given suggestions at the moments of most intense pain, will be found very helpful.

The simpler suggestions are, the better. Short and epigrammatic sentences are most effective. The patient should be given three or four of these to be used at the hours prescribed by the operator. They should be simply short, definite affirmations of improvement. Auto-suggestions to be used upon retiring at night might be something like this: "I am going to sleep soundly", "I shall wake up much stronger", "The pain will disappear", "Such and such a symptom will trouble me no more."

Similar suggestions may be used at meal-times if digestive disturbances are feared or at any other time of day when desirable. The operator must use his own judgment in dictating the suggestions to be used. One excellent method of using auto-suggestion is in connection with water drinking. It has been stated previously that attention should be given to seeing that the patient drinks the needful supply of water each day. Very many people suffer from nothing so much as the effects of too little water taken internally. Patients may be instructed to drink three or four glasses of water daily at stated times, not too near meals, and the act of drinking may be made the occasion for very valuable auto-suggestions. Tell the patient to drink the water slowly, with each swallow or sip repeating appropriate statements like the foregoing, but having special reference to the water that is being consumed. The thought should be that the water is going to stimulate the digestive functions, remove the causes of disease and tone up the system generally. Under proper instruction from the operator, patients will derive great benefit from this method.

In the preliminary examination of each patient, the operator ought to learn all possible about the habits of eating, drinking and sleeping formed by the patient; and when he detects anything that should be corrected, he should use the corrective means as a vehicle for suggestion. Nine patients out of ten will be found to err in the matter of taking too little liquid and taking it at improper times. The less liquid taken with meals the better, and the more pure water taken at other times, within reason, the better. The method for a patient to use in giving himself auto-suggestions varies according to different authorities. Some regard it as only essential to repeat the suggestions "parrot-like" as it might be expressed, a large number of times. The advocates of this theory believe that the repetition is all that does the work.

On the other hand, I have found best to instruct patients to give themselves auto-suggestions after the following manner Compose the body in a sitting or reclining position for a few minutes and strive to compose the mind at the same time as much as possible. By that I mcan tranquilize the mind as much as possible and to this end it is best to close the eyes and to select a quiet place for the preliminary rest. Then repeat the suggestions two or three times mentally in a quiet, determined way, using the will to enforce the subjective obedience. Some patients have told me they secured the best effect by imagining the subjective mind to be a separate personage to whom they addressed themselves in a tone of command. Then having given the suggestions, banish the whole matter from the objective mind as much as possible and go about the ordinary duties of life, simply strong to keep a cheerful and untroubled frame of mind. If the thoughts revert to the matter at all, simply reaffirm the suggestions and again turn the mind from the matter. If there is pain, reaffirm the suggestions against it every time it occurs. The theory of this is, of course, that the subjective mind, having once grasped suggestions given in this way, will go on repeating them subconsciously, and acting upon them unless they are controverted by stronger adverse suggestions. Thus auto-suggestion consists in giving good suggestions and refusing to allow adverse ones to gain a foothold. Right at this point it may be well to give a caution to all operators and patients. I have just said that we must avoid adverse suggestions as well as inculcate good ones. No point in the whole practice of Natural Healing needs to have greater stress laid upon it than that. Instruct all patients to say nothing to others with reference to their treatment.

Patients should not discuss their ailments nor their treatment with people outside their own near relatives, and not with them if they are opposed to mental therapeutics, either through ignorance or prejudice. Well-intentioned persons who do not understand the laws upon which Natural science is based will often times create an atmosphere of adverse suggestion which no efforts of operator and patient combined can possibly overcome. Even the Savior Himself more than once said ta those whom He had healed, "Take heed ye tell no man.'"

We can understand no other reason for such an injunction except that in His complete knowledge of the subjective powers, He realized that adverse suggestion might overthrow the structure that faith and His own masterful spirit had built up. Most certainly no good can come from skepticism and "throwing cold water" upon faith and hope, and if there were no deeper reason for it than that, an atmosphere of doubt and cynicism ought to be avoided by the patient. Even if the theory of the subjective entity were a fallacy, it never yet helped a sick person to tell him he was worse or was going to be so, or that the means he was using to get well were useless ones.

Avoid adverse environment and atmosphere whether you believe in Natural Healing or not. Don't discuss the treatment with the idle or the curious nor approach it yourself in any but an earnest spirit. It is an insult to the power and the God within us to indulge in idle chatter and frivolous gossip about so vital a matter.

THE LAW OF NATURAL HEALING

CHAPTER V

Absent Treatment in Theory and Practice

AUTO-SUGGESTION THE BASIS OF ABSENT
TREATMENT – FAILURE TO UNDERSTAND ABSENT
TREATMENT THE REASON FOR OPPOSITION TO IT -
INFLUENCE OF HEALERS PERSONALITY – TELEPATHY -
ANIMAL MAGNETISM - SUBJECTIVE SUGGESTIONS

The discussion of auto-suggestion leads naturally to the consideration of its application to cases other than those in which it is used as a means of treatment supplementary to the efforts of the operator himself. Autosuggestion forms an important part of all absent treatment.

Probably no aspect of Natural Healing is more liable to misconception than is the treatment of the sick who are resident at a distance from the operator. Absent treatment is no new thing. It has formed a part of many systems of healing heretofore, though it has almost always been assailed with criticism and not infrequently with derision. This, however, is the result of a misconception of its principles. It is evident that all direct suggestions must, in one sense, become auto-suggestions before they can have curative value.

In other words, they must be received objectively before they can be acted upon subjectively, and so, while received from an external source, they are "auto" or self applied suggestions when they reach the subjective mind. This being the case, it is evident that distance between operator and patient has no effect upon the possibility of imparting suggestions. It merely affects the potency which they will have. That is to say, a suggestion sent in a letter is just as good as one given by word of mouth, barring the consideration of the giver's personality.

THE LAW OF NATURAL HEALING

If a patient can be convinced of the value of self-given suggestions, and can be persuaded to apply them systematically according to the operator's directions, he will get as much good from absent as from direct treatment.

The percentage of cases that can be helped by absent treatment is in general likely to be smaller than that benefited by direct treatment, because comparatively fewer patients can be found in whom it is possible to inculcate subjective faith without the aid of the operator's personality. Those patients in whom subjective faith can be implanted as the result of acceptance of the suggestive theory can be treated as well absently as in the operator's presence. It must be remembered that in treating absently, the patient is deprived of what should be the most potent of all suggestions, viz., the operator's own personality. Just what constitutes "personality" is of course a thing most difficult to define, but I believe that it is, in effect, the ability to transfer suggestions subjectively. Heretofore we have considered suggestions as having objective origin exclusively. But it is my belief that certain minds have the power of transmitting suggestions from subjective entity to subjective entity without objective intervention. That is, the transfer is subconscious on the part of operator and recipient. It is probable that all human minds have that power to a degree, but that those persons in whom this attribute is most strongly marked are those of whom it is customary to speak as "magnetic" or "possessing strong personality."

The phenomena of telepathy or "thought-transference" have been investigated far enough by strictly scientific experiment to show beyond a reasonable doubt, that subconscious minds do communicate one with another. In these communications, material space is of no moment. Therefore, I believe that in treating by Natural Healing methods, objective suggestions are constantly supplemented by subconscious emanations from the operator's subjective entity, and the operator

31

who most strongly influences patients in this way is the one who is most successful and, in common terms, is said to possess the most powerful personality. It is well said that almost every settled belief of mankind, no matter how wild and chimerical it may have become in the course of years, has had some basis of real fact from which it originated. Probably the strongest proof of immortality lies in the instinctive belief we all have in it, and in like manner it is probable that the very existence of any deep-rooted general belief, though it be manifestly an erroneous one, is an argument for its origin in truth.

So great a number of people believe in what is known as animal magnetism as a curative agency that I am inclined to think that there really is some basis for belief in it. I think there must be some emanation of the human mind to account for the faith, which is so widespread, in the theory that one person can impart a healing magnetic current or current of nerve force or energy to others.

I have no doubt that the many patients who ascribe their course to the animal magnetism they suppose I possess have really been cured by the class of suggestions I have been discussing. All I claim is that anybody else could impart the same force if he had trained his subjective entity to the work for a sufficient time. I do not deny that many of the cures attained by Natural Healing methods are almost miraculous in their nature when viewed from a standpoint outside the knowledge of Natural laws, but they are miraculous in exactly the same way as a steam engine is a supernatural creature in the estimation of a savage. An untrained mind could not build the engine nor heal the sick, but properly trained it can do either. I consider that it is by systematic training in the use and practice of objective suggestion that the mind becomes capacitated for giving subjective suggestions of the kind I have been discussing.

CHAPTER VI

Subjective Methods

USE OF SUGGESTIVE SUGGESTIONS – ATTITUDE
TOWARDS PATIENT PREVIOUS TO TEATING HIM –
SUBCONSCIOUS CONTINUANCE OF TREATMENT –
WHAT THOUGHT IS – PRACTICAL METHODS IN ABSENT
TREATMENT – EXAMPLES OF ITS EFFECT

I have made it a practice since I became aware of this
telepathic potentiality which I believe exists in the subjective
entity, to strive to direct it toward the treatment of a great
number of cases. For instance, as soon as I am summoned to a
new patient who is confined to his house, I seek to find out as
much about the circumstances of the case as possible, the nature
and duration of the trouble, and so forth. Then, before going to
the patient, I sit down alone in quiet and make my mind passive,
directing it to the patient I am to see. I make a mental picture of
the patient and of his condition of disease, setting my will to
work against the unhealthy condition that exists. I try to force my
subjective mind to precede me to his bedside and to begin the
work of preparing his subjective forces to rally to his physical
aid. In the same way, I keep in mind at certain hours of the day
all patients who need to have me do so, during all the time I am
treating them. After every examination of a new patient, I adopt
this method and I am confident that this telepathic
communication is set up between me and many of my patients to
their material benefit. Once having secured such a subjective
connection between the minds of the operator and patient, it is
not unreasonable to believe that the subjective suggestions first
given are repeated again and again indefinitely. A pebble thrown
into the ocean, physicists tell us, creates a wave motion that
would go on forever into infinite space if the water extended so
far, and in the same way I believe that a suggestion once set in

motion goes on repeating itself till stopped by an insurmountable barrier of adverse force or is recalled by its sender.

In my own experience with cases treated absently, I have found certain methods valuable, and these I will set down at this time, but students will find a wide field in this connection for the exercise of their own ingenuity and inventive resources. It cannot be too often repeated that every individual case must be approached as though it was the only one of its kind that ever existed. Experience may prove the value of general methods, but their indiscriminate application to special cases must be carefully guarded against. It is, in general, harder to secure the confidence of a patient whom you are going to treat absently than that of one to whom you can talk and thus form your own impressions of his temperament and physical needs as well as impress him with your own ability to help him. This being the case, I have usually found it valuable to write to the patient somewhat at length, in the first instance, setting forth the power of the human mind to communicate with its fellows subconsciously or telepathically. Naturally all this has to be done in a manner and in language suited to the person you are addressing. You should explain that your highly trained mind can come in contact with the patient's mind and stimulate it to the performance of its duties in regulating the physical health. You can impress him with the fact that you are going to teach him how to help himself. The wireless telegraph instrument which is actuated by the mysterious wave in the ether produced by its twin instrument many miles away, may be used as an illustration of the results which you are going to produce. A great many of the best scientists of the day believe that thought is simply a wave motion in the ether not dissimilar to the waves which produce light, magnetism and electricity.

The patient should be instructed that in order to secure the good effects from such communication between his mind and yours, it is necessary not only that you should send him these helpful suggestions and forces, but that he should be at the same time prepared to receive them. Consequently you should appoint certain periods of the day, from ten to twenty minutes in length, during which times the patient is to devote his whole attention to the treatment. Previous to receiving the treatment, the patient should retire to a quiet room and in solitude recline or sit at ease for some minutes, relaxing the body and mind as completely as possible. The eyes should be closed and the attention fixed upon the thought of the coming treatment, and upon the fact that curative forces are to be received from the operator. At the precise moment indicated for beginning the treatment, the patient should place one hand upon the back of the neck at the base of the brain, and the other either over the seat of the disease or at the base of the spine. Then during the time of treatment, the mind should be centered upon the receipt of telepathic force from the operator, and the patient may be directed to imagine, if possible, the force entering the hand which is upon the location of the disease and so passing through the system to the other hand. Many patients so directed will actually feel a sensation of mild tingling as from a gentle galvanic current.

Of course the patient understands that during the periods when he is following the above instructions, the operator is concentrating his mind upon the case and is devoting the energy of his will to imparting the curative force. That this method is helpful in a great variety of cases cannot be doubted, for I have seen it exemplified in my practice too often to question it for an instant. I remember one case in which I sent the patient, a lady who had suffered years with rheumatism, an ordinary copper cent, with instructions to hold it firmly upon her forehead during the time of treatment. I suggested to her that the force would, by reason of her fixing her mind upon the coin, enter her body through its mediumship. This suggestion took effect so strongly that within two weeks after the receipt of the coin, she wrote me that the copper became so hot during the treatments that she could not retain it in her hand! But what was of the only real importance in the case, her rheumatism disappeared within a month after beginning the treatment and did not reappear, though she had been practically crippled with it for years.

In another case, the wife of a prominent physician in a southern city applied to me for absent treatment for an internal tumor. She could feel the force which I suggested she would feel, in a marked degree. She described it as similar to the sensation of mild electrical treatments. She never failed to feel it during the periods prescribed for treatment but could feel it at no other time, though I finally discontinued concentration upon her at the times set, because I felt confident that the subconscious repetition would go on in her mind exactly the same, as indeed it did.

Now I have no doubt that some will consider the sensations these patients experienced to have been pure imagination, but the fact remains that one was cured of rheumatism and the other found the tumor materially decreased in size with every indication of its ultimate absorption without the surgical operation that was at first declared to be necessary to save her life. Whatever the theory of any student or reader may be, these results, coupled with equal successes in many other cases, indicate to my mind that there is a force within us that can heal our bodies if we only get hold of the way to set it at work. The method of subjective suggestions as outlined above is of course to be supplemented by the use of such helpful suggestive formulas as have been indicated in a previous chapter for the self-help of patients treated directly. All the usual methods before outlined, including water-drinking and general hygienic measures may of course be as well made a part of absent treatment as of any other. Suiting the means chosen to the case in hand is the secret of success.

CHAPTER VII

Acute Conditions

WHEN DRUG MEDICATION IS NOT ONLY RIGHT BUT NEEDFUL – WHEN NATURE NEEDS HELP – FORCES DISREGARDED FOR YEARS CANNOT BE BUILT UP INSTANTLY – FALLACIES OF SO-CALLED SCIENCE – NATURAL HEALING IS COMMON SENSE – WONDERFUL RESULTS OF A YEAR OF PRACTICE

In previous chapters I have outlined a general system of treatment in accordance with the theory of Natural Healing. I have emphasized the facts that suggestion is the basis of all curative power and that the ingenuity and tact of the operator must guide him in the selection of suggestions to be used and in choosing the method of applying them to individual cases. In presenting brief general instructions for diagnosing certain diseases, and directions for treatment, I have no intention of laying down hard and fast rules for the student. I intend simply to show how I have treated certain cases successfully. By no means, however, do I mean to claim that other methods of procedure along the lines of Natural Healing may not be quite as efficacious. However the treatment may vary in details, the principles laid down in previous chapters must be rigidly adhered to. Let the operator gain his patient's confidence, create subjective faith in the treatment and secure the cooperation of the patient, and success is certain as sunrise after dawn.

It may be proper, before proceeding to the treatment of diseases, to call attention to one point which might otherwise confuse the student. It will be noticed that I do not attempt the cure of acute disease conditions by Natural Healing methods, I have always been the advocate of stomach medication, within limits, in acute conditions arising from the action of germs or bacilli. The reason for this is in perfect accord with the theories I have heretofore advanced. An acute attack of a germ disease is not a functional disorder. The germs of disease are noxious organisms and are to be combated like any other pests or vermin. Because I am a believer in the power of the subjective mind, there is no reason resulting from that belief to prevent me from attacking potato-beetles in my garden with Paris green, plant-lice in my conservatory with tobacco fumes, or rats in my domicile with strychnine. Just in the same way, when my human tenement is infested with bacilli, it is perfectly reasonable to aid nature to be rid of the vermin by killing them. It has been shown beyond question that certain preparations of drugs are able to destroy certain disease germs by poisoning them to death. Such drugs the physicians term "specifics" for the diseases in question. It is therefore perfectly proper to administer these drugs in sufficient quantities during acute attacks of germ diseases in order to assist Nature to kill the germs.

This does not at all disregard or belittle the fact that Nature would, without the drugs, summon the subjective forces and cast off the germs. A perfectly well-nurtured and well-developed human frame would recover from any germ disease in time, unassisted by drugs, but these crises invariably come on suddenly, and, in the average person, Nature cannot rally the subjective forces quickly enough to destroy the invading germs before they have overcome the vitality and destroyed life. In a person of perfect development and vitality, the struggle between the life forces and the invaders would be a protracted, bitter and painful one, but the vital force would conquer in the end, if no specifics were used. Very few human constitutions, however, are fitted for such a struggle unaided. Every human organism would possess the requisite vitality and stamina to withstand these sudden incursions of the enemy if the subjective forces had been trained from infancy or early youth. It is the lack of knowledge of the forces within ourselves that makes the human frame subject to disease at all. Had the subjective forces of a man been trained from earliest youth, he would not only possess a physical development practically invulnerable to germs of disease, but in the event of an attack occurring through some unusual circumstances.

Nature would be able to summon the subjective forces instantly to the point of attack and medicine would be needless. We cannot, however, put off the subjective education till a crisis is upon us and then build up in an hour the neglected structure of years. Therefore in acute attacks, medicine ought always to be resorted to. Once, however, the acute stage has been passed. Nature reasserts itself, the subjective forces if properly directed, again coordinate the functions and convalescence ensues. During convalescence from an acute attack, suggestion is vastly better than any other ciu-ative agency. And as I have before stated, in all cases where a chronic state has resulted from the continued derangement of the functions, it is the only means to permanent and complete recovery. In exactly the same way, it is ridiculous and even criminal to treat the acute stages of injuries to the body by suggestion alone. Some cults of so-called scientists and others profess to treat fractures of bones and similar conditions solely by mental means. Such a procedure is not only grossly nonscientific, but worthy of all censure. Natural Healing makes no such pretensions for the very reason that it is scientific and based upon natural laws and not upon superstition or magic. Suppose the bone of the arm is fractured. There is no attribute of the subjective mind which makes it natural or likely that any force will be exerted to replace the portions of the fractured bone in position. There is no bodily function concerned in such a procedure nor is any provision made for such a contingency.

True, when a fracture occurs, the subjective forces are immediately directed to the seat of the injury and a fluid is exuded from the ends of the fractured bone which will cause it to knit or cement itself together if the ends are in juxtaposition, but this process would take place just as surely if the ends of the bone were twisted through the circumference of a circle as though they w^ere in their natural position. Therefore it is necessary that they should be placed in their proper relation to each other by mechanical means before the natural process of repair is allowed to take place.

Once the bones have been placed correctly with relation to each other and held in that position by suitable appliances, Nature will perform its proper function of renovation, and at this time the progress and efficacy of the work can be hastened vastly by the right use of suggestion. There never was a remedy or a theory in the world that could not be run into the ground by too anxious endeavor to make it fit unnatural conditions. The student may rest assured that the theory of Natural Healing is unassailably correct, but like every other good and perfect thing, it must be applied with common sense.

In the same spirit of intelligent application of Natural truths, we must recognize that every operator will find cases in the course of his practice that he cannot seemingly benefit or cure. In a certain year of my practice, carefully kept records of every case I undertook revealed the fact that nearly eighty percent, of my patients, many hundreds in number, expressed themselves as materially benefited or entirely cured. The remaining twenty per cent, included such patients as did not voluntarily express themselves as to the results of the treatment, together with those others who took only one or two treatments and made no report whatever upon their subsequent condition. Of this latter class, I have heard in indirect ways from several who were completely cured and hence had no further need to come to my office. Still I have no doubt that there was a certain small percentage who received no benefit they could perceive. That fact does not by any means assail the value of Natural Healing.

CHAPTER VIII

Some Popular Misconceptions

SEEMINGLY MIRACULOUS CURES NOT ALWAYS AN
ADVANTAGE - SUPERSTITION STILL EXISTS – TRYING
TO SIT UPON TWO STOOLS – OPPOSING THE OPERATOR
YET HOPING FOR HELP

Any exponent of a system not universally understood is
certain to meet with opposition. Sometimes it is the active
opposition of the unbeliever, sincere or otherwise, and more
often it is the opposition of ignorance that will not consent to
receive the benefit the operator is anxious to confer.

A great many patients look for sudden and seemingly
magical cures. It is almost invariably that class of cures that is
bruited abroad most widely. It occasionally happens that a severe
case of a dangerous malady will be cured by Natural Healing
agencies in only one or two treatments. This simply means that
the patient so cured has happened to be especially suitable,
temperamentally, for such a success, and also that the operator
has succeeded in securing the necessary subjective attention in
shorter time than is usually required. Such an outcome of a case
is to be explained simply upon the lines of what has been said
before with reference to temperamental make-up and the
securing of co-operation between patient and operator.

But to a portion of the public it seems miraculous. The
fame of the operator goes forth more like that of a magician than
that of a healer applying a purely scientific remedial agency. The
result is that scores of people who have not the slightest
comprehension of their own vital forces, rush to consult the
operator, expecting to be healed instantly by some hocus-pocus
worthy of the darkest days of superstition. There may not be a

single case among them capable of such an outcome as attended the original case. But if the healer does not cure every one of them in an instant, despite their ignorance and half-concealed disbelief, they are prone to brand him as a fraud. Always strive to impress patients with the fact that it takes time to build up the forces they have long neglected and been unaware of.

In a certain number of cases that I have remarked, patients have stopped taking treatments after what they considered to be a fair trial, resulting as it seemed to them only in slight benefit. Afterwards, however, their condition constantly improved till complete recovery ensued. This I consider to have been the result of subconscious continuation of the treatment. The suggestions given during the treatments had begun to have their effect and the subjective forces once set in motion, continued the good work after the patient had objectively ceased treatment. For this reason, I always urge patience and persistence in treatment even though immediate results be not fully up to the sufferer's hopes.

I have no doubt that occasionally the very belief in the possibility of a miraculous cure is a most potent suggestion and may in some cases be strong enough to effect just that result, but nine out of ten who approach the subject with any such superstitious or ignorant attitude toward it, are half-doubtful after all and so get nowhere. They are too far emerged from superstition really to believe in anything miraculous, but they are not sufficiently enlightened to grasp the real significance of subjective phenomena, so that their small knowledge is a disastrous thing and, between two stools, they sit upon neither.

This is the class of patients who do nothing to aid the operator and who rather hamper him than otherwise by their secret attitude of opposition. Most of such patients labor under the delusion that they are laying themselves liable to the imputation of weak-mindedness by having anything to do with such a method of healing the sick. At heart they are superstitious and ashamed of it, not realizing that the deepest truths of exact science are concerned in the attempt to cure them. They can believe in a science that typifies itself in a sugar-coated pill, but a science that deals with the human soul is an undreamed-of element in their philosophy. I have known patients to approach the subject of mental therapeutics in the same spirit in which they would consult a clairvoyant, palmist, fortune-teller, or other vulgar fraud; that is, with an air of shamefaced bravado, fearful lest some one should see them enter the office! Is it wonderful that such as these should require some little time to learn whereof they speak and to harmonize themselves with eternal truth?

But let a patient place himself unreservedly in the operator's hands, seek to follow his directions implicitly, and, in short, faithfully to comply with Natural laws, and he cannot fail of benefit.

CHAPTER IX

How to Succeed

THE OPERATOR HIS OWN BEST SUGGESTION - ATTITUDE TOWARD PATIENTS - RIGHT LIVING - HEALTH IS BEST WHEN FORGOTTEN - EMOTIONS REFLECTED IN PHYSICAL CONDITIONS - COST OF WRONG THINKING - SELFISHNESS THE ROOT OF ALL ERROR

The operator should always remember that he himself is perhaps the most potent of all suggestions to a patient. He should never betray any anxiety or uncertainty about a case and should never under any circumstances allow a patient to perceive that he considers his condition less favorable than on some previous occasion. It often requires very great self control to prevent a patient from getting unfavorable or discouraging suggestions in this way. A sick person is frequently much more keenly observant than a well one and instinctively he watches the countenance of the healer or physician for an indication of his real condition. It is the operator who makes his own personality the strongest suggestion for good that wins the greatest success.

It is always best to tell a patient in a cheery tone that he is looking better than it is to ask him how he feels. Some patients feel it a part of the duty incumbent on ill-health to reply to such questions in a mournful and deprecatory tone, seeking for bad symptoms and admitting improvement grudgingly. Needless to say, this attitude is a producer of unnecessary adverse suggestions, and should be nipped in the bud when possible. A good, cheery suggestion is better at any time than an inquiry which in itself admits of a doubt as to improvement. The preservation of health is something that is of vital interest to everybody, but only too frequently the very carefulness that it engenders defeats its own purpose. How many people do we meet whose whole minds are centered upon the minor ills and ailments of life and whose sole thought seems to be the apprehension of physical illness. There are of course certain essential rules of hygiene which need to be observed in order to maintain physical health, but beyond them, the very best attitude that can be taken toward physical conditions is to forget them.

If people will attend to securing proper nourishment, fresh air, sunlight, out-of-door exercise and bodily cleanliness, they need to have no further thought with reference to the condition of the body. A proper regard for the above elements of physical well-being is ennobling and uplifting to the mind, but a petty, fussy care and constant fear of incurring ill from the ordinary experiences of life, is useless and hurtful. People who are in a perpetual ferment over the danger of taking cold, inhaling noxious germs, eating unwholesome substances, catching some sort of infection wherever they go or in otherwise incurring some dire evil that exists largely in their own imaginations, never have any peace of mind, and in time degenerate into petty, small-minded, selfish and self-centered beings who are alike a trial to themselves and to those with whom they come in contact. What they need to learn is that the physical health demands proper care but less attention. Take the proper hygienic precautions with reference to the body, then let it alone. Examining the state of the health every hour of the day with the object of striving to find flaws in it, is like setting out a choice plant in a garden under all favorable conditions for its growth and then pulling it up daily to see if its roots have sprouted and taken hold upon the soil!

Forgetting one's self is one of the best rules for human happiness that was ever laid down. The person who lives from within outward has an estimable advantage over the one who lives from without inward. A self-centered man is always an unhappy one because his sphere is so extremely small! And the longer he fixes his attention upon himself as the sole object worthy of notice in the scheme of creation the smaller his object of adoration really becomes! The selfish man is always a petty one. He does not think with anybody but himself and there has been quite an appreciable amount of thinking going on in the universe, in all probability, outside of his own entity! But the unselfish man lives from within outward, and he thinks with the best of his fellow men, and so comes to think with the Divine Intelligence as well.

It is well known that the evil passions which animate the hearts of human kind exercise a direct chemical action upon their physical structure. Noted scientists have gone so far as to analyze the perspiration and the saliva of men strongly under the influence of the passions of rage, revenge, jealousy, etc., and from these tests, without other knowledge, to determine what one of the emotions named had possession of the subject at the time. For every one of these passions defines itself in the formation of its own particular poisonous substance in the physical excretions. Who has not seen the victim of raging anger or grief almost prostrated, with wildly beating pulse, high fever, and racking headache after a paroxysm of such emotion? How many cases of apoplexy and death have resulted from giving way to unbridled wrath, often over absurdly trivial matters?

On the other hand, what physical well-being and manifest enjoyment of living is to be seen in the form and face of the man whose life is calm and well-regulated, and full of good will and good deeds toward his fellow men. That virtue is its own reward is true as Holy Writ, but not in the pessimistic sense in which the saying is most often quoted. It is true, because no man can do good toward his fellow men without reaping the largest portion of it himself.

Evil passions cost him who harbors them more than they cost the object of them. It has been well said that revenge, of all human feelings, promises more than any other and repays the least. It promises its possessor the keenest of pleasure, and it turns into ashes in his hand the moment he has attained it. And all the course of its pursuit is but blowing upon the embers of a flame that consumes the heart in which it rests.

"I'll get even with him," is often heard uttered by a person who has suffered a real or a fancied injury. No doubt the saying will come true. It can happen in two ways: either you will repay the injury in kind and so you will be even with the aggressor by lowering yourself to his level; or you will requite it with kindness and, in the language of the Scripture, "heap coals of fire upon his head" until you have raised him up to yours. Probably the latter method will actually furnish the most satisfactory returns, unless you prefer the lower level for yourself. Selfishness is the root of all error, and ignorance is the root of all selfishness. The ignorant man hopes to better himself by thinking of himself alone, and therein lies the whole reason for the errors of our lives.

PART II

CHAPTER I

Diseases and Their Treatment

ADAPTING THEORY TO PRACTICE – DIAGNOSIS – WHY
SPECIAL CASES ARE OUTLINED – RHEUMATISM –
CAUSE – SYMPTOMS – TREATMENT – TYPICAL CASES –
PATROLMAN'S CURE – HOW ADVERSE SUGGESTIONS
WORK – NEURALGIA – SCIATICA

The treatment of various diseases by Natural Healing requires less variety of method than most systems, because the theory of suggestion implies general, rather than local treatment in most instances. It is the operator's first aim, after having stilled whatever acute pain may exist, to build up the general system of the patient, arouse his latent forces and direct the power that is within him to eradicate all physical conditions which make disease possible. Since this is true, there need never be any fear of applying the whole practice of Natural Healing to any specific case, within the limits that ordinary good judgment should define, and the operator has no need of any very complicated system of varying his treatment to suit different diseases. It is, nevertheless, well to adopt certain methods of applying the general practice in a variety of ailments; and in the following chapters I shall aim to outline the devices which I have found most satisfactory in the course of my own work.

Details of actual cases are given in order that they may furnish the student with types by which he may judge methods and results. Brief directions for diagnosis of cases may also help some students and readers. It is, of course, impossible for very many who may be able to do effective work as Natural Healers, even to attempt the making of expert diagnoses. But an intelligent knowledge of the symptoms of ordinary diseases will be found essential. There are certain physical conditions which indicate definite physical causes, and recognition of these will be necessary to the operator. It very often happens that patients believe themselves to be suffering from ailments entirely different from what they really have. If an operator can disabuse a patient of such an impression, he has already gone far toward getting his mind in proper attitude to receive help. A sick person who can be made to regard his sickness in really correct perspective is rare, and it is almost always true that he exaggerates the discomfort and danger of his condition. It is therefore necessary for an operator to be able to form a just estimate for himself of the real gravity of a case in order to do the best work. The operator should avoid, however, allowing his anxiety concerning his patient to be reflected in his face or tone, and he should especially guard against allowing an atmosphere of doubt or despair regarding a case to permeate even his own mind, lest subconsciously it be reflected in the mind of the patient.

At best, only a few general symptoms of the common diseases can be given, but it is hoped that they will be enough to guide the student in making right conclusions in this portion of his work. Experience and the study of proper reference books are the only two means to gaining an ability to make correct diagnoses. Students should not make the mistake of attempting the treatment of acute conditions, for reasons that have been explained. Nature cannot rally its forces quickly enough to combat a fever or any such crisis, unaided, but once the crisis is passed, the forces of suggestion can be brought into play to great advantage. Perhaps one of the most frequent diseases which the student will be required to treat is RHEUMATISM.

No ill that flesh is heir to more thoroughly illustrates the truth of what has been said about the medical treatment of disease. The great majority of rheumatic cases become chronic, and no medicines known will cure rheumatism after it has become a settled condition, but I have cured the disease in chronic stages in a large number of cases. It takes time, to be sure, but I know of no other way of curing it except by methods of suggestion. Rheumatism frequently originates from taking sudden cold, contact with damp ground or residence in damp swampy localities. It is sometimes ushered in by a violent acute condition in which the patient is taken suddenly with very violent pains in the joints accompanied by high fever. The joints swell rapidly and are almost unbearably sore to the touch. After the fever has subsided, the disease frequently becomes chronic and there is more or less constant pain and swelling. If this condition becomes a settled one, after many months or years, the joints become permanently set and often badly twisted or distorted. This is caused by the hardening or destruction of the synovial fluid of the joints and the roughening and inflammation of the membranes lining them. This condition is practically incurable by any means.

The synovial fluid when wholly vanished or changed into calcareous deposits, cannot be restored any more than the punctured ear drum or the amputated limb. Nature makes no effort to effect such a restoration. However, before this final stage is reached, it is possible to set restorative forces to work by means of which the circulation can be made to carry off the impurities which cause the condition and check the ravages of the disease. The cause of rheumatism is claimed by many to be uric acid in the blood, produced by non-digestion and poor assimilation of food. At least, an acid condition generally accompanies it.

It should be noted that the acute condition called rheumatic fever occurs in only a comparatively few cases, and unless this appears at the outset, it is perfectly proper to use suggestive methods at any stage of the disease. Rheumatism may be distinguished by the dull, grinding and often occasional nature of the pain, together with the swelling of the joints and the puffed appearance they present, as well as the location of pain in them. Rheumatism also settles in the muscles in some instances and is then called muscular rheumatism; or in the sciatic nerve, when it is known as sciatica.

Neuralgia is a rheumatic condition locating in the nerves and is paroxysmal in nature and excruciatingly painful. When it locates in the facial nerves it is known as tic-doloreux. The treatment for rheumatism should begin with thorough but gentle examination of the parts affected and the usual passes and vibratory movements made to secure the patient's attention, with the object of relieving whatever pain may exist. As soon as the patient is relieved so that he can be interested, the operator should explain what he plans to do, namely, eliminate the conditions which produce the disease by arousing the patient's own inward forces. All success depends upon getting the cooperation of the patient and making him understand the principles that have been outlined heretofore. Then, securing the patient's attention by fixing the eyes steadily upon his, proceed to arouse the solar plexus and stimulate the digestive functions as before directed. Explain to the patient that as you pass the hand over his body and affected joints, the circulation will be stimulated and directed to the parts, thus absorbing and bearing away the impurities to be eliminated from the body by the natural channels. At the same time, the stimulation of the solar plexus will arouse the activity of the digestive and excretory organs to take care of the burden the blood is to bring them. Instruct the patient to drink large quantities of water, not less than three quarts daily, in order to assist the natural process of elimination that you are about to set up.

When the rheumatism is in the lower limbs, it is very often possible to effect a complete cure in the first treatment by seizing the proper moment when the patient's attention has been secured and fixed upon the affected part and ordering him in a firm tone to lay aside his cane or crutch and walk. Assure him that he can do so without pain or discomfort, and that when he has done so, the pain will not return. In a large majority of cases the result will be that the patient will walk off without help and will declare himself greatly improved. The second treatment will often put such patients so far on the road to convalescence that nothing further will need to be done for them. Nature will take care of the process of renovation and elimination from that time on.

All the time a patient is being treated, it is of course necessary for the operator to fix his mind firmly upon the fact that he is going to help the patient, that the patient is going to be better, must be better. One must always intend to do a thing before he can do it, and so a fixed, definite intention to cure the special case in hand should always be the operator's attitude toward the patient. The best practice is to explain to the patient as you go along the object and intention of each portion of the treatment. It engenders his confidence alike in the operator and in the treatment, and it aids in directing his attention to the affected part. This very attention is what will send his subjective forces to work there, equalizing the circulation and stimulating the cells to eliminate and recuperate. A case of the type mentioned above came to my notice some time ago. Patrolman Wm. R. R of the Worcester police force was stricken with rheumatism in a very painful form. It settled in his feet and they swelled badly and made it impossible for him to wear his shoes or to appear on duty.

He came limping to my office to be treated, though he had manifestly little hope of relief. I made the usual examination, told him what I was going to do, and stimulated the necessary centers. Then after vibrating the feet slightly, I told him I had cured him; that he could put on his shoes and go out. He did so and before the day was over the swelling had practically disappeared. There was a slight recurrence on the second day after, but a treatment promptly overcame it, and he had no further trouble. This was a typical case where the patient's attention and the operator's intention combined to produce a condition in which the surprise of a command to "walk out, cured," turned the scale from sickness to convalescence.

The case of Frank G. S , of Spencer, Mass., showed that the same forces can be set to work in the same manner, even when the disease is of long standing. Mr. S had been crippled with rheumatism for a number of years, but though he was bent over as the result of it, his joints were not set. I first went to his house to treat him and found him on crutches. After a few minutes' treatment, I suddenly commanded him to walk out of doors, for I had seen that I had secured his attention and that the very suggestion of my expected visit had prepared him for a cure. He walked out without crutches, after some demurring, and joined in the sport of some children playing about the yard. The following day he came to Worcester and walked perhaps one-third of a mile over city pavements without trouble. Gradually the subjective forces began to overcome the effects of the long-standing condition and he steadily improved. In the course of his convalescence he came in contact with some one who opposed his progress with adverse suggestions, and for a time he did not improve, but after that influence was overcome, the advance toward health continued.

One of the greatest difficulties always to be encountered is the adverse influence of those who are most sincerely interested in the patient. Strange as it may seem, those nearest to a convalescent patient, both by kin and affection, are often those who retard his recovery most. They may not understand the method by which he is being helped or it may run contrary to their preconceived ideas, but they surround the patient with an air of incredulity or amused ridicule which is fatal to his progress. Doubt and the fear of being thought weak-minded or credulous invade the patient's mind and swiftly undo all the good that the operator can attain in many treatments. It is strange that the most loving of relatives and friends frequently value their own opinions and prejudices higher than the health and welfare of those near to them, though they would be shocked and indignant were any one to tell them so.

NEURALGIA is one of the most painful forms of disease known, and results, like other rheumatic troubles, from exposure to cold and dampness, and from the effects of drugs or stimulants which affect the nerve tissue. The cause of neuralgia is very frequently found in the stomach, though often local interference cause certain sets of nerves to be affected. Neuralgia may be generally diagnosed by the shooting or streaming nature of the pain and its spasmodic recurrence. Inflammation accompanying neuralgia is different from that of rheumatism when it is present at all, though neuralgia is not always accompanied by inflammation. A neuralgia that has been of long duration and become settled in a certain set of muscles is known as neuritis, though the term is most properly applied to neuralgia affecting the ulnar nerve.

Neuralgia is best treated by passes over the affected parts accompanied by strong suggestions intended to still the pain. Vibration at the base of the brain is often effectual, and, as in all cases, the general treatment should be commenced at once in order to start the process of renovation. The patient generally will be found to be eating too much food and drinking too little water.

SCIATICA is one of the most painful forms of rheumatism or neuralgia. It seems to partake of the nature of each. The pain is most, excruciating and follows the course of the sciatic nerve from its point of emerging from the body, down the back of the legs to the feet. A patient so afflicted is unable to walk and suffers greatly. Medicine is not found to have any very beneficial effect. Very often surgery is resorted to and some extremely rigorous expedients have been resorted to, like opening the patient's leg and stretching the nerve by mechanical means.

The mind, however, has the power to cure sciatica without any of these horrors, and in a number of cases which have occurred in my practice, I have succeeded in relieving and finally curing it, by the simplest suggestive means. Mr. C , a business man of Grafton, Mass., about thirty five years of age, was a great sufferer with sciatica. He came to me one morning in much pain and I treated him by placing one hand upon his shoulder and passing the other along the course of the affected nerve, while I informed him that the circulation would now be stimulated and the pain would cease. He went away relieved and felt better nearly all day, but at night was taken violently ill with sickness at the stomach and much pain in the affected leg. He had to have an opiate administered. In the morning, however, the pain ceased and he came to me. I treated him once more, and told him the sickness and violent pain were just what he needed and what I had expected he would have. From that time on, he had no more pain, the soreness disappeared, and he has had no recurrence of the trouble though that was a year ago.

His case was one in which it was possible to arouse and set working the subjective forces in a short time, and I believe the severe experience he had at night was simply the result of Nature's supreme effort to throw off the disease. It is to be noted that those patients who exhibit strong nausea and a violent paroxysm of the trouble a few hours after the first or second treatment, may almost infallibly expect to experience sudden and often phenomenal cures. When the Natural forces make so sudden and so strong an effort to throw off diseased conditions, the effort is usually very successful.

THE LAW OF NATURAL HEALING

CHAPTER II

Nervous Derangements

THE AMERICAN DISEASE – TOO FAST A PACE – CURE FOR NEURASTHENIA – HYGENIC REGULATIONS – LUMBAGO – MR A'S TYPICAL CASE – POLICEMAN I CURED OF LONG STANDING LUMBAGO

No disease, not even excepting tuberculosis, is so common in this age as is the ailment known as nervous prostration or nervous exhaustion. It is often termed "The American disease" from its great prevalence in this country, and from the fact that its origin is supposed to lie in the high tension of life in America. It is characterized by a great variety of symptoms and may lead to the most serious consequences. It is regarded as being the outcome of over-stress placed on the nervous system together with insufficient nutrition, resulting in a deterioration of the fiber forming the nerve sheathes. It is a condition that results from a long continuance of its causes, and consequently is one that requires a lengthy period of recuperation.

Its symptoms are far too many for enumeration and vary greatly in each individual case. In general, there is lassitude, emaciation, indigestion and dyspepsia, oftentimes vertigo and heart palpitation. Inability to fix the mind on work or study, feeling of complete bodily exhaustion, depression of spirits, and a great variety of different symptoms, some of which almost border on hallucinations, mark the disease. If unchecked, it may develop into softening of the brain and insanity, though many cases simply degenerate into a state of chronic invalidism which lasts for years or for life.

Nervous prostration or neurasthenia is a disease that can

be cured only by a long and faithful course of treatment. It is no use for a patient to look for a magical or miraculous cure as the result of two or three treatments. Physicians will admit that there is no medicine known which is of any use in this trouble. If they do not openly admit it, they do so tacitly, from the fact that the many sanitariums devoted to its treatment do not resort to medicine at all except for other ailments existing at the same time. Neurasthenia can be cured only by a long course of recuperative effort on the part of the Natural forces coupled with an abolition of the causes which have brought on the condition. The patient must abstain from whatever has been the cause of the condition, be it over-work, improper diet or indulgence in habits of drug taking. Not even in rheumatism, is there so much need of copious water drinking as there is in any severe nervous disorder. A nourishing diet, consisting largely of milk and cream if they can be taken should be insisted upon. Regular out-of-door exercise is essential and a general outdoor life is very beneficial.

If these hygienic regulations are attended to strictly, recovery may ensue in a long course of months without any other treatment. In ordinary medical practice, that is all the hope that is held out to patients. Nature is simply left to repair by the slow process of time the ravages made in the nerve structure. Natural Healing, however, offers the only known method of shortening this period of recuperation. It does not neglect the proper direction and control of the Natural forces as does every other system. The policy of letting recovery drag along with no stimulation of the curative forces is like an attempt to get up steam in a boiler with the fires all banked and the dampers shut tight. The methods used by the Natural Healer stir up the fires, and turn on the forced draught, so that the engine proceeds to work anew with vital force and pressure behind it.

The treatment for nervous prostration should be unremitting. The general treatment of stimulating the centers and the functions is the most important and should be carried on systematically every day. All the resources of auto-suggestion and self-help for the patient should be brought into play, and suggestions to combat the feeling of despondency which characterizes the disease should be constant. It is safe to say that the time of recovery from nervous prostration can be reduced fifty per cent, by careful attention to the general theory of suggestion. The operator needs to take the patient's case right upon his own shoulders and use every expedient, objective and subjective, that will tend to direct the sufferer's own mind to the recuperation of his nervous system.

Once the patient's confidence is secured, the work of recovery is begun and it will progress with gratifying celerity. The general bodily health will be found to improve, and as it does so, the patient's progress will be increasingly rapid. In this day of vast numbers of nervous sufferers, operators thoroughly understanding the treatment and cure of the disease will find fruitful and lucrative fields of practice. They will render untold service to their fellow men and will reap substantial rewards for themselves.

LUMBAGO is a painful affection that not infrequently precedes and ushers in sciatica. It is of rheumatic origin and results from a debilitated condition during which the patient happens to fall victim to a severe cold. The cold settles in the back m the region of the lumbar vertebrae. There is much soreness and pain across the small of the back and not infrequently the patient believes himself to be attacked by kidney trouble. There is often great difficulty in straightening up, spasms of pain seizing the patient as he strives to do so. If neglected or not checked, the pain and soreness is frequently communicated to the sciatic nerve and all the excruciating discomforts of severe sciatica develop.

One typical case of lumbago in my practice of several years ago I remember particularly. Mr. C. S. A , a well-known merchant of Worcester, was attacked by lumbago and suffered severely for some time before I was called to attend him. I went to his place of business and found him just able to keep about, every movement giving him great pain. I determined on rapid procedure, for his first words were to the effect that he did not believe I could help him. I held his gaze for a few minutes, firmly willing that he should give me his confidence and be helped. Then, suddenly, I passed my hands twice down his back rapidly and firmly.

"Straighten up," I ordered, and he did so. "Bend far over," was the next direction and he obeyed without demur or difficulty. "You are cured,'" I said- and he was! Another treatment removed the soreness from the back and there was no recurrence of the trouble. Patrolman Henry Laviolette of the Worcester police force was also a sufferer from lumbago, and for a long time was not able to stand up straight and walked with much difficulty and pain. With him I adopted a not dissimilar course, for I considered the initial impression made by the recommendation of a friend who sent him to me to be sufficient to establish confidence or '"rapport." I scarcely touched him, but almost instantly ordered him to lay his cap on the floor and pick it up again, which he did to his own great surprise, as he declared he could not stoop half way to the floor without agony when he entered the room. After a few manipulations, he was able to turn and twist his body in any manner without great discomfort, and in the course of brief subsequent attention to his case, I completely removed his trouble, which has not recurred during the several years that have elapsed. Strong will and intent to cure, together with self-confidence on the part of the operator; confidence secured and subjective faith engendered in the patient; this is the secret of curative success.

THE LAW OF NATURAL HEALING

CHAPTER III

Subjective Suggestions

WHAT ARE THEY – SUBJECTIVE RELATIONSHIPS –
SUBTLE FORCES OF THE MIND – REMARKABLE
INSTANCE OF TELEPATHIC COMMUNICATION – MISS
L'S STRANGE EXPERIENCE – HOW THE HEALER
ASSUMES HIS PATIENT'S ILLS – EXAMPLES IN MY
PRACTICE

While it is true as I have stated so emphatically in the foregoing chapters, that the force which cures is within the patient himself, yet the subtle relationships which may come to exist between the minds of patient and operator are worthy of the greatest consideration and they may form an important factor in effecting cures. The two minds must be in harmony with each other of course, according to the basic theory of Natural Healing.

If the mind of the operator cannot exert the right influence upon the patient's subjective entity, the latter cannot be stimulated and taught to realize its benign potentiality over the physical being. When the two mentalities are in harmony or "en rapport" as the French expression happily puts it, the subtle and elusive relationship that exists between them furnishes one of the most interesting fields of investigation for the reader. Some curious instances of this relationship may prove interesting to students, though I cannot say they are valuable except as they show how the establishment of this harmony reveals itself in cases where real success is obtained. One of my patients, Miss M. L, a lady of nearly middle age and decided intellectual ability, had suffered a considerable length of time with nervous exhaustion, she being naturally of a neurasthenic temperament. She took a number of treatments at my office and showed herself a willing and intelligent patient. She was already acquainted with many psychological principles and it was not a difficult task to instill the requisite subjective faith and to convince her of the efficacy of the treatment. After being treated some little time and receiving an appreciable amount of benefit, she went to a country resort one hundred miles away for a vacation period. The incidents which followed were told me by the lady herself, and of course I had no other objective knowledge of them. I had, however, been interested in her case and had determined that my mind should continue to be in touch with hers in order that she might lose none of the good effects of the treatment she had been taking.

Every day, during the four weeks she was absent, the lady assured me, I appeared to her at certain hours, and treated her. The phantasm, if such it is to be called, would appear generally when she was walking alone or in company with others, or when sitting out-of-doors. At such times it would apparently give her treatments in the exact manner I had been accustomed to in my office. There was no objective anticipation of the manifestation on her part and she was greatly surprised and puzzled over it, not to say terrified, when it first occurred. She first thought it purely imagination and strove to dismiss it as nonsensical. Later she began to be seriously disturbed lest her brain might be affected, but as a matter of truth, there never has been the slightest reason for such an explanation. The appearance of the manifestation was hard to describe, she said. In general it had the appearance of myself, but it was something felt rather than objectively seen. It never withstood the scrutiny of objective vision. Still she was fully conscious of its presence at various hours which had no regularity of recurrence, and she was sure she was always keenly alive to all objective impressions at the times in question. At length she began to dislike the manifestation and grew almost morbid over it, setting her will strongly against its recurrence, whereupon it soon stopped appearing. Soon after, she returned to her home, resumed regular treatments and was finally very materially benefited.

Now, I am perfectly frank in saying that, except casually, I did not think of the patient in question while she was absent. But I had very firmly impressed it upon my mind previous to her going away that my treatment should lose none of its force while she was gone; that the improvement should be continuous and that my subjective suggestions should go out to her all the time she was gone. I have said that I firmly believe in the subconscious repetition of suggestions by minds trained to that end, and I am confident that my intention was so strong that it actually manifested itself in the manner related. Of course this is an exceptional case, but it illustrates the unfailing power of suggestion when once set in force, according to my belief. It will be noted that the manifestation repeated itself under all sorts of circumstances until she herself willed that it should not do so further. The suggestion went on indefinitely till turned back by a stronger adverse one.

Occasionally, though fortunately that is not commonly the case, the operator finds that he takes on for a short time at least, some of the symptoms of his patients. I have treated a few cases where this was so, but I think no operator ever need be afraid of such a thing doing him material injury, for if he is strong enough to assume the burdens of another, he is strong enough to throw them off. I never had any lasting ill-effects from such a cause, yet some of the instances of which I speak are curious and may be of interest. It has occasionally happened that in treating cases of neuritis or of swelling and inflammation resulting from strains or injuries that I have felt exactly the same muscles affected as the patient complained of. This condition never persisted more than a few hours, however. In one instance I remember, the patient, a Mr. M , about forty-five years of age, was troubled, among other things, by a difficulty in controlling the action of the kidneys and bladder. It became a source of the most constant annoyance to him, and when I was called to see him it was the first thing I strove to alleviate. I proceeded in the usual manner to stimulate the general nervous system and digestive functions, and then made a few transverse passes across the region of the kidneys with the express purpose, as I told him, of strengthening the retentive powers of the urinary tract. To my own great surprise, I was immediately seized with a very unusual activity of the kidneys, which made itself unmistakably noticeable to me.

I had very strongly willed him to be relieved in that respect and here again the remarkable harmony that can be made to exist between minds showed itself. Of course the experience was only temporary with me, while with him there was no subsequent recurrence of his trouble. He was cured of it at once. From that time on his general health improved. Just previous to my visit to him, he had fallen to the ground four times in a single day as the result of vertigo attendant on his condition. Afterward he was able to go about the streets alone with considerable freedom. I have no doubt that time will witness his complete restoration to health.

CHAPTER IV

Asthma

CAUSE IS NERVOUS AND DIGESTIVE – RELIEF BY
ABOLISHING CONDITIONS OF CAUSE – BRONCHITIS –
DIABETES MELLITUS – RECOGNITION OF NATURAL
HEALING BY OLD SCHOOLS IN TREATING DIABETES

A disease very common in New England and prevalent everywhere. It is evidenced by irritation of the mucous membrane of the lungs and bronchial tubes. It is a disease that originates in a great variety of causes and seems to be the result of nervous and digestional disturbances. It is very distressing, the patient being unable to breathe except with the greatest difficulty, and when its spasmodic attacks are at their worst, the sufferer shows all the symptoms of strangulation.

The effects of damp climate, cold, irritation of stomach, lungs and other organs, over-study or excess of mental activity, suppressed functions and other causes are alleged to produce asthma. Asthma is almost invariably accompanied by constipation, and it is not at all improbable that the infection of the blood arising from this condition is the real producer of the disease. Considering this fact, I have always aimed to relieve the constipation by strong abdominal stimulation and suggestions to overcome the tendency to intestinal inaction. Then I suggest strongly to the patient that the circulation is to be quickened and amplified in the bronchial region so that the irritation of the tubes will be diminished.

If temporary relief can be given in this way for a day or two, as it almost always can if the suggestions are properly given; the relief of the constipated condition then begins to work a real relief in the irritated membranes. Asthma necessarily takes some little time to cure, for there is a considerable process of elimination to be gone through with in a chronic case, but the most stubborn of cases can generally be cured in this manner. Patients should be encouraged to take outdoor exercise and to the observance of a diet that will preclude the return of the constipation.

BRONCHITIS is another ailment characterized by inflammation and irritation of the bronchial region. It generally begins in an acute attack and becomes a chronic condition later. Its symptoms are akin to those of asthma, but not generally so distressing. Bronchitis, however, is sometimes the fore-runner of tuberculosis of the lungs and should not be neglected for that reason aside from its annoying and troublesome symptoms. The constipation which is generally sure to exist, in tendency at least, should be relieved first and then careful stimulation applied to the base of the brain and to the bronchial region. The suggestions should be toward increasing the circulation and the nervous energy, especially that of the sympathetic nervous system, as the functions of breathing and circulation are so nearly connected with the bronchial region. Out-of-door air and water drinking, and in fact all hygienic precautions which tend toward elimination should be prescribed in all conditions which are marked by inflammation of the mucous membrane or other tissues.

PLEURISY or pleuritis is characterized by sharp cutting pains in the chest and depressed feeling. It is often accompanied by fever, and in the acute condition is often violent and dangerous. The pain finally becomes chronic and recurs whenever the patient takes cold or is exposed to sudden changes of the weather. The treatment for pleurisy is the stimulation of the nerve centers of the chest region and general circulatory stimulation. The mechanical suggestion of magnetized water is often helpful in pleurisy. Some operators may find gentle manipulations of the patient's shoulders and body, which have a tendency to limber up the muscles in the chest region, a helpful suggestion. Anything which will increase the blood supply in the outer tissues will be likely to decrease the pain.

DIABETES MELLITUS is one of the most common ailments affecting the kidneys. It is marked for purposes of diagnosis by the presence of sugar in excessive quantities in the urine and is regarded as being caused by an improper action of the liver which does not change over and prepare for assimilation the saccharine products of the food in the proper manner.

A striking and gratifying thing to every student and practitioner of Natural Healing is the fact that it has now come to be recognized by some of the most prominent specialists in the treatment of diabetes as the best possible method of coping with the ailment.

In a recent article, John Duncan Quackenbos, M.D., a famous physician and member of many learned societies, says, "Diabetes mellitus has been added to the list of diseases curable by intelligent suggestion, a number of cases having been successful treated. Diabetes implies an error in the metabolic activity of the liver cells, whereby the sugary elements hurry through that organ unchanged or are produced there in excessive quantity to be excreted by the kidneys instead of being retained in the system and converted into energy. The rationale of suggestion here involves assurance of psychic control over the manufacture and assimilation of sugar; the ordering of its retention in the body, and its transformation there into capacity for work and happiness; the destruction of the appetite for the carbohydrates, together with the intense thirst characteristic of the disease, and creation of tolerance and even desire for the prescribed diet; directions to insure an equable increase in flesh, strength and activity. Diabetic patients respond immediately to such an appeal; and no better illustration of psycho-physical control can be adduced than the disappearance of this functional disease in obedience to the decree of the trans-liminal self."

In another portion of the same article he says: "The present attitude of reputable science toward intelligently administered and wisely guarded suggestion as a therapeutic agent is thus incontestably one of hearty approval and support. The world's deepest thinkers accept its truths and construe its facts."

Shorn of all its technical language, the description of the treatment of diabetes by suggestion, as given by Dr. Quackenbos, is exactly the course I have used and here recommend to the student. The stimulation of the liver and colon in the usual manner is accompanied by suggestions to promote the process of sugar disintegration and assimilation by the liver cells. The suggestions are given in the form of assurances that the liver can cope with any form of diet and have no difficulty in so doing. There is no need to advise water drinking in this case, for the almost abnormal thirst which accompanies it will assure the patient getting fluid enough. Suggestions are often valuable to assuage this thirst and give the patient relief from its discomforts. It is certainly gratifying to observe the adoption of Natural Healing methods by the leaders of the regular schools, whose rank and file are often found arrayed steadfastly against anything that is not bounded by the limits of a pill or a potion.

CHAPTER V

Epilepsy

SYMPTOMS – TREATMENT – EXPECTANT ATTENTION
ILLUSTRATED – EPILEPSY CURABLE BY NATURAL
HEALING METHODS – MISS K'S CASE

A nervous disease commonly known as "fits" or the "falling sickness." It is characterized by the strange contortions and foaming at the mouth with which the victim suffers during the paroxysms of the disease. The fits, are always heralded by a peculiar scream which the victim gives as he falls and which cannot be mistaken once having been heard. There is always a great rush of blood to the head; frothing at the mouth and unconsciousness, during which the body is badly distorted and the limbs twisted in uncouth convulsions. The only thing to be done in the presence of one of the attacks is to lay the patient in as comfortable a posture as possible with the head slightly raised and prevent his doing himself an injury. A rolled handkerchief or a stick covered with soft cloth may be put between the teeth to prevent biting the tongue.

The treatment of epilepsy must necessarily be of general nature and of faithful continuance. An entire systemic change must be undergone before a complete cessation of the attacks can be looked for. Still a gratifying decrease in the frequency of the attacks can be looked for from the early part of the suggestive treatment if it is properly administered.

The patient is prone to live in constant dread of an attack and very often to invite one by his expectant attention regarding it. The mind can be turned in a new channel in the early stages of the treatment and the courage of the victim aroused to combat the recurrence of the attacks so that they will really be decreased in frequency. One amusing illustration of this fact came to my knowledge in a railroad train in this state. The gentleman who related the circumstance was not a practitioner of any kind, but he was a man who was not easily excited in an emergency and was gifted with a fund of good common sense. He was riding about his business one day in a train when he observed a young man obviously ill at ease and discomposed.

Finally the young man accosted the gentleman in question with the following words, "I am sorry to trouble you, but I am an epileptic and I am going to have a fit- I know I am! Will you take care of me?" with each word becoming more and more excited. "Certainly," said the gentleman coolly, "I'll look out for you, but you're not going to have any fit today- in fact you couldn't have one if you tried. Now go ahead and have anything you want, if you can, I'll take care of you!"

This attitude struck the epileptic as so ludicrous that he burst out laughing and in a few minutes was seated comfortably and talking animatedly with his new-found friend. He had no fit and when he left the train was profuse in his thanks, saying he had not had so pleasant a day for a long time. In all probability, the least betrayal of anxiety at the time he thought himself about to be taken ill would have precipitated a severe attack. The phenomena of expectant attention are often responsible for a great many human ills. All the resources of the general treatment, especially stimulation of the brain and nerve cells, acceleration of the circulation and careful attention to the condition of the digestive functions should be resorted to in the course of treatment for epilepsy. No medicine known will cure this disease, but properly applied suggestion has been known to restore many sufferers to health.

One of the cases of epilepsy I have met in my practice was that of Miss K , who resided in a Worcester County town. She had been a sufferer for a number of years with the malady and exhibited all the symptoms, including frequent violent fits. She was unable to go anywhere with any peace of mind as she was constantly afraid of falling in one of the paroxysms. She took a course of treatment for several months, the object of which was to renovate the nervous system. One of the most gratifying early results of the treatment was the increase in confidence she experienced in going into public places. She was finally able to attend the theater, church and other public assemblages with almost no fear, and the number of attacks in a given period decreased notably. The progress of the case was slow, but it appeared that once the subjective forces were set in motion, there was a constant tendency toward improvement and ample ground for hope that in the end the malady would entirely disappear. It is a difficult thing to persuade some patients to persist long enough in the treatment to secure a complete cure. In all nervous diseases, time must be allowed for Nature to rally its forces and the average sufferer has not the ability to wait patiently for a necessary period to elapse. Where nerve tissue is deteriorated, nothing but the slow process of Nature's own ordaining, quickened by the proper Subjective stimulation can make good the damage, and it is rare indeed that Natural processes of repair are more rapid than the ravages that produced the condition.

CHAPTER VI

The Root of Many Ills

CONSTIPATION – ITS CAUSES AND EFFECTS – ELIMINATION ONE OF THE MOST IMPORTANT FUNCTIONS – ILL EFFECTS OF CATHARTICS – PROPER TREATMENT BY NATURAL HEALING METHODS – PILES OR HEMORRHOIDS

Constipation may be confidently pointed to as the primary cause of about one-half the ills of which patients complain. The cause of constipation is the failure of the colon or larger intestine to produce the peristaltic motion of the membrane which lines it in the natural way and at proper times. This motion is the function of the tiny papillae or folds in the lining of the colon and tends toward moving the waste matter of food through its natural course to the point of elimination from the body. The colon has also an absorbent power of great importance as is shown by the instances in which patients have been kept alive for long periods solely by food administered through its agency. It is plain that when the waste products of food are not properly eliminated by the colon, the many organic poisons, ptomaines, etc., with which the waste material is laden, are absorbed into the system and turned into the blood supply together with the healthful products of food, to poison the whole stream of life. That this is exactly what happens when the bowels do not perform their natural fimction at least once daily, cannot be doubted. Therefore, it is fair to say that at least fifty per cent, of the ills that are ascribed to impoverished condition of the blood are really the result of constipation.

84 THE LAW OF NATURAL HEALING.

When the blood is poor, the nerves and muscles are not

properly nourished and even the brain cannot get its necessary renovating material. Scarcely a nervous patient was ever found who was not troubled seriously with constipation. The constipation once become chronic, it and its effects become intro-active and the very nervous and blood deterioration it causes, aggravate the disordered condition of the digestive function.

The act of eliminatmg the waste products of food is governed by the same nerve system that controls the other functions, and the normal desire to perform this function is automatic as that of breathing. It is however necessarily governed by the will, and when the intimation of nature that the function should be performed is not obeyed promptly, the peristaltic motion is checked and retroverted, and in a short time, it becomes inactive. Lack of proper exercise, preponderance of certain kinds of food, lack of attention to the calls of nature either

through want of opportunity, neglect or false modesty, will all cause constipation, and in fact practically all people of sedentary life or nervous temperament are more or less its victims.

The use of cathartic drugs is one of the most deplorable habits into which a person afflicted with constipation and its attendant ills can be led. Nearly all the cathartics, and even the aperient salts in large quantities, are poisons ; and in order to perform their effect, they have to be absorbed into the blood and carried to the membranes of the intestines, since their action depends upon the stimulation of the peristaltic motion by increasing the amount of liquid excreted by the surface membranes of the intestines. A portion of these drugs is of course not eliminated and as it soon becomes the fact that larger and larger doses are needed to produce their effect,

THE LAW OF NATURAL HEALING. 85

the blood soon becomes laden with poison which is perhaps even worse than the natural poisons sought to be rid of. Drugs are a delusion and a snare in the treatment of constipation

and if persisted in will work the worst possible harm.
But since the function of the intestines is governed by
the solar plexus, or "abdominal brain/' which controls all the
vital machinery of the body, the methods of Natural Healing
which are directed in great measure to the co-ordination of
the forces which actuate the nervous centers, are particularly
efficacious in combatting the effects of impaired digestion and
elimination.

If, by the usual expedients of suggestion, the subjective
forces can be directed to the stimulation of the solar plexus,
the action of the stomach, liver and small intestine will be
quickened, the natural secretions of the colon will be amplified
without recourse to the cathartic poisons and the peristaltic
motion will be resumed in the due course of time.

Very often it has been proved in my practice that the use
of water prepared in the manner indicated in a previous chapter
is the best possible suggestion for the relief of a constipated
condition. Sometimes the relief is experienced very quickly
after the beginning of the treatment and in other cases the
progress is more slow, but if persisted in, the most stubborn
case will yield to suggestive influences. And when the
constipation
is cured, the operator will find, in a large percentage
of his cases, that the ailments and diseases which the patient
complained of when he first applied for treatment, have vanished
also.

Once having conquered the condition, of course the patient
must so conduct himself as not to relapse by reason of the
same neglects or indiscretions that produced it at first. Outdoor
exercise and a varied, proper diet should obviate all
danger of recurrence.

86 THE LAW OF NATURAL HEALING.

PILES OR HEMORRHOIDS

are the direct and most painful results of chronic constipation.
They are the most common of rectal ailments and result both
from the infection of the tissues by unexcreted poisons and

from the unnatural distortion of the rectal muscles and tissues caused by straining in the effort to produce natural movements. They are of numerous kinds, such as blind, bleeding, protruding, etc. Fistula is the extreme stage of the diseases in which the tissues are actually eaten through and others than the natiu-al orifice exist. In all cases, piles are curable only by the removal of the cause, which is constipation. The process of renovation may be a slow and discomforting one, but once having cured the cause, the diseased condition of the tissues will disappear in due time.

CHAPTER VII

Paralysis

CAUSES OF SHOCK – HEMIPLEGIA – PARAPLEGIA –
CREEPING PARALYSIS – TREATMENT - CIRCULATION
RENEWED – CONSTIPATION TO BE GUARDED AGAINST
- IMPORTANCE OF ENCOURAGEMENT TO PARALYTICS -
FACIAL PARALYSIS - TWO NOTABLE CASES - LOSS OF
VOICE - MISS D 'S REMARKABLE RESTORATION OF
SPEECH - MISS K AND MISS R

Paralysis or "shock" as it is commonly called, is the result of blood clots lodging in the brain and oppressing certain of the centers there so that the portions or functions of the body they control are rendered useless. The cause of such blood clots is occasionally external injury, but much more frequently impure blood and sluggish circulation, the result of constipation or other allied causes. The attacks come on suddenly and without warning and the victim is generally stricken from comparative or seemingly complete health to a most pitiable condition of helplessness. There are many kinds of paralysis, and some "shocks" are so slight as to affect but a very small portion of the body, or any one of the senses, the power of speech, etc., while others render the whole body or half of it useless.

That form of the trouble which affects one side of the body is called hemiphlegia, while paraphlegia is the term used to denote paralysis affecting the lower portion of the trunk and limbs. Another form is known as creeping paralysis, in which the initial shock, frequently a slight one, is followed by a slow progression of the effects, larger and larger areas of the body being affected gradually. Paralysis agitans is the "shaking palsy" of old time terminology. In this form the patient is unable to control his muscles at all and the limbs quiver and shake in the most distressing manner. Facial paralysis generally affects but one side of the countenance at once and is an annoying form of the trouble for it robs the face of expression and generally gives it a ghastly or repulsive expression aside from affecting the speech and frequently the eyesight.

In all cases of paralysis, the stimulation of the circulation is the first essential. Constipation must be carefully guarded against and every means used to restore a normal quality of the blood and induce an accelerated circulation. In some cases the deterioration of the circulatory function has gone so far that nature cannot rally her forces sufficiently to overcome the trouble, and unaided, she practically never does so. Unless the methods of Natural Healing are used to set the curative powers of the mind at work, the patient almost infallibly suffers subsequent attacks which terminate his life, though they may not occur for months or even years after the first. If taken immediately after the first shock, however, the circulation may be so improved as to absorb and remove the cause of the trouble and the process of repairing the damage done made to go on in natural course.

The basic idea of treatment for paralysis is of course always to remove the source of the trouble by general treatment, but the patient generally wants immediate relief from his inability to use his limbs. Passes over the affected portions accompanied by strong suggestions relative to increased power of locomotion or use of the limbs in various ways will generally be found to give immediate relief. Nothing encourages a patient suffering with paralysis so much as to make him do things with his arms and legs that he has not been able to do, or believes he has not, since he was stricken. He is helped in the best sense by such encouragement because it engenders the necessary subjective confidence in his ultimate recovery and sets his own mind forces to work to help him unconsciously to himself. Too often patients suffering in this manner become utterly despairing because of their inability to do as they had previously, and the very depression that ensues hastens the progress of their trouble. Therefore the operator can conscientiously try to impress the patient with the benefit he is deriving from an ability to move about more actively, when as a matter of fact, that consideration is secondary to the real object of the treatment, viz., the removal of the cause of the condition. Anything which makes the patient think he is getting on well is the best influence he can possibly have about him.

In the course of my practice I have had some very interesting cases of paralysis; and those in which the ailment has been taken early enough in its course and the patient has been willing to comply faithfully with the requirements of treatment for a sufficient length of time, have exhibited pleasing results. Two cases of facial paralysis I recall were so much alike that they may be mentioned together. Mr. A. C, a man in middle life, and a mechanic by occupation, was suddenly stricken with a paralysis which deprived him of power over one whole side of his face. He was entirely without expression on one-half of his countenance, while the other was normal in appearance. I was called to him within a few weeks after the attack, and as he was a healthy man of active habits and sufficient vitality to warrant the belief, I concluded he would be easily cured. I treated him two or three times by passes made over his face and by strong suggestions that he could control the muscles in the affected part. In stimulating the brain centers the intention was of course directed to the opposite side of the skull from that on which the trouble was located, from the well-known fact that the halves of the brain govern opposite sides of the body.

It took but a short time to direct the subjective forces toward the affected nerves and muscles in the patient's face and soon he could move the one side as well as the other. All of the effect the patient cared for was the renewing of his normal expression and control over his facial muscles, but the real object lay deeper and was attained through the favorable attitude the patient's view of the matter caused him to take toward the treatment. I have no doubt the cause was wholly absorbed and eliminated by the circulation, since he has had no recurrence of the trouble whatever in many months.

Mr. Frank D , a cigar-maker, was the other unfortunate spoken of. His trouble was of longer standing, but he was a younger man than the former patient. His case was a severe one, and not only was the side of the face set and mask-like, but the eye muscles were also affected so that he could open and shut his eyelids only by lifting and lowering them with thumb and forefinger. When he went to sleep at night he was obliged to close his eye in this manner. His condition was not only disfiguring, but very annoying, and there were fears expressed that he might become much worse affected so as to lose possibly his sight and hearing. I pursued exactly the same course as in the case previously spoken of. I made the eye the point of attack, and when I had succeeded in getting the patient so he could govern its opening and closing in the usual way, he was overjoyed. In a very short time, he had no further difficulty with the eye and has had no noticeable effects from the trouble since the conclusion of the treatment.

LOSS OF VOICE is said to be one of the most difficult of all physical ills to cure. It is generally found to result either from a paralysis of the throat and vocal cords or from the after effects of a severe cold or throat trouble of the grippe or influenza type, in which case it is probably a condition of systemic poison. Catarrhal conditions also may cause loss of voice, but this generally predicates a destruction of some portion of the vocal apparatus, and is most likely to be incurable. Three very notable cases of voice restoration in the course of my practice come to mind. They were all cases of long standing and seemed to have been caused by colds, or throat affections of that nature. All three were cases of complete loss of the power to utter a loud sound. The patients could simply form the positions of speech with the tongue and lips, but nothing but the faintest whisper would answer their strongest efforts to make themselves heard. This condition had in each case persisted for a number of months.

The first of the three cases to be brought to my attention was that of Miss Helen D , the daughter of a well-known Boston business man. The loss of her power of speech followed after a severe attack of cold and sore throat. It was believed at first that she would overcome it in a short time, but as she did not, medical advice was sought. A number of specialists treated the young lady, at considerable expense, but to no good. The loss of voice had persisted for nearly a year and a half, when the case was brought to my attention during a visit of the young lady to a relative in this city. I realized the difficulty of the case, and while I of course betrayed no doubt of the matter to the patient, I told her relatives confidentially that I felt there might not be any great success, owing to the possibility of destruction of some portion of the vocal apparatus. However, I gave the patient two treatments and informed her that within forty-eight hours after the second one, her voice would return to her. This I strongly suggested to her and I exercised the most determined intention to produce just the result I promised her.

In short, it was a case where it was worth while to risk everything on a single cast. On the evening of the last day included within the time set, the young lady and her aunt attended a performance at the theater. In the midst of the performance, the young lady suddenly found, with a feeling of the utmost amazement, that she could speak aloud. She kept trying her voice under cover of the music and applause, being careful not to let her aunt know of her recovery lest the surprise should upset her. When she left the theater and returned home she greeted the other members of the family in her natural tones, and since that time, months ago, she has no difficulty. I have always considered this case as one of the most dramatic proofs of suggestive influence I ever heard of.

The fame of this case brought me two others of similar nature, both young ladies, one of whom was a well-known public singer in Holyoke, Mass. The first of the cases, a Miss K , began to gain in voice strength with the first treatment. Her progress was constant and gradual, and she finally resumed full powers of speech without any sudden change in her condition.

The second case, that of the singer. Miss R , was of the opposite nature. She had lost her voice, like the other two patients, as the result of a severe cold. She came to my office and took a series of treatments lasting a number of days. She seemed to experience but very little benefit and finally she left for her home. Less than a week after she arrived there, I received a letter from her full of the most profuse gratitude and stating that on the second day after her return from Worcester, her voice came back to her almost instantly, and she was then in full possession of it. In a few weeks afterward she was able to resume singing and has not so far as I know ever experienced any further difficulty.

CHAPTER VIII

After Effects of Injuries

WHEN NATURAL HEALING PLAYS ITS PART – LIVED
WITH HIS NECK BROKEN – CASE OF EDWIN PARLIN A
MARVEL TO MEDICAL SCIENCE – FRACTURED FOURTH
VERTEBRA – GIVEN UP TO DIE AFTER MANY MONTHS
IN HOSPITAL – CURED IN TWO WEEKS BY NATURAL
HEALING METHODS – A NOTABLE TRIUMPH – CASE OF
JOHN J BURNS

Very often treated in the most advantageous manner by
Natural Healing methods. Convalescence in any physical
condition can be quickened materially by the skillful
suggestionist and particularly where the convalescence depends
upon the renovation of injured tissues by Natural means. In cases
of burns, fractures, sprains, bruises, cuts, contusions and injuries
of all kinds where nature ordinarily repairs the damage, the
process can be hastened wonderfully by properly directing the
subjective forces. Of course no renovation at all would ever take
place if the subjective forces did not compel it, for what is
referred to as "Nature" in this connection is of course nothing
but the subjective mind of man which has his physical
well-being for its normal task of guardianship. Natural Healing
is in the last analysis nothing more than the proper direction
of the natural forces within the patient's own being, to the
exercise of their normal duty.

In cases of physical injury, as has been indicated
heretofore, the aid of surgery is first to be called into play.
Broken bones must be properly set, cuts cleansed and sewed up
and wounds of all sorts attended to, according to the procedure
appropriate to their kind. The subjective forces cannot unite a
broken bone in a minute nor heal a cut instantly nor reduce a

sprain in the twinkling of an eye. They were never intended to do so, and it would be supernatural if they did. But having used the proper mechanical means to place the injured parts in as near as possible their proper relation to each other, nature begins the work of repairing the damage forthwith.

Then the stimulation of the natural impulse of renovation is the province of the operating suggestionist, and his work will do what no other branch of the healing art can do, that is, shorten the time usually taken to repair the damage done to the physical being. In cases of strains and bruises where there is no actual severing of tissues as in cuts and fractures, I know that the cures by Natural Healing methods are so much quicker than those by any other as to appear almost miraculous. And in the same manner the period of convalescence from other serious injuries is frequently so much shortened by a competent operator as to excite wonder and admiration. Perhaps one of the most remarkable cases in the whole course of my practice, at least the one which has at various times been given the widest publicity, was that of Mr. Edwin Parlin of Worcester. Mr. Parlin was a man above fifty years of age when he passed through one of the most peculiar adventures that ever falls to the lot of mankind. He was employed at the Grove Street Works of the American Steel and Coke Company at the time when an extraordinary accident made him one of the most famous patients in whom medical science has taken an interest in recent years. He is famed as one of the very few men who have fractured the vertebrae of the neck and survived. Probably he is the only man whose complete recovery of health and strength after a fracture of the cervical vertebrae has ever been recorded.

During the evening of August 29, 1900, Mr. Parlin, who was in his own home, took a small hand lamp with a glass chimney, and started down the cellar stairs, in the pursuit of some domestic employment. He never performed the errand upon which he started. His shoe caught in some manner upon the top stair and he fell headlong to the bottom. Strangely enough the lamp with its fragile chimney was not injured in the least, but when Mr. Parlin was picked up it was discovered that his neck was broken. The fourth vertebra was not merely dislocated but broken as well, and the fragments were pressing upon the spinal cord in a manner that is usually declared to be fatal without a possibility of recovery. There was much hemorrhage and altogether it was a case in which by all precedent the patient should not have survived till the physicians could reach his side. Mr. Parlin's head was twisted upon his neck in the ghastly manner of one who has died by hanging, but still a spark of life flickered in his breast.

He was a man of fine physique and vitality and it was determined by the eminent surgeons who had been attracted by the report of so notable a case, that an operation should be attempted. He was etherized and the effort was made to set the broken vertebra. This was finally done and Mr. Parlin emerged from the effects of the ether to find himself utterly helpless below the chin. It was as though his body did not exist at all, for he was unable to move a single muscle or to realize a single sensation in any portion of his being below his head. For three weeks the patient lay in this manner, rapidly losing flesh and apparently merely awaiting the end of his sufferings. Then the attending physician tried to turn the sufferer slightly in bed and the neck broke again. The process of knitting together of the bones had not gone far enough to stand the strain of the movement and the result was a return to the condition of things immediately after the accident. The process of resetting was gone through again and by this time it was judged wise to take Mr. Parlin to the city hospital. The task of removal was finally accomplished, and then there began a series of trials of every expedient known to medical science to restore him to health. All the time he seemed to be wasting away and soon grew to be scarcely more than a skeleton. There was no return of sensation or muscular power to his body or limbs, and it seemed impossible that he could long survive. Massage, electricity and every other expedient, mechanical and medical, that was available at the hospital, was tried; but after many months of apparently absolute stagnation in his condition, Mr. Parlin's case was given up and he was sent home to live or die as the case might be, with the ultimate fatal end of his sufferings seemingly but a short time removed.

It was after the unfortunate man had been a month at home, gaining not a whit apparently, that I was called into the case. I went to see him and a more pitiable sight never met my eyes. There he was in bed, lifeless below the chin, and unable to do more than to turn upon me the most appealing, hopeless gaze, while the tears ran unchecked down his cheeks. I am frank to say that I doubted if any power on earth could help him. Certain as I was and am of the wonderful forces Nature has invested us with, I doubted if in this sad case they could be aroused soon enough to save the sufferer. But I pitied him so I determined that if will of mine could save him, he was to be saved. I threw every bit of will-power and intention I could muster into the effort to set his subjective forces in motion. I told him in the strongest terms that I would help him, and I passed my hand two or three times from his shoulder to his wrist along the arm next me as he lay in bed.

I was with him but five minutes at the outside, but for four or five hours following my visit, he felt the first sensation in his arm that he had experienced since his accident. His arm tingled and throbbed and it seemed as though the circulation and nervous energy were coming again to the member. The following day, at about the hour of my visit on the previous one, Mr. Parlin suddenly called out to his wife in great excitement. She was alarmed and came hastily to him. He begged her to remove the bandages with which his arm was swathed and when this had been done, to their great wonder and joy, the shrunken and claw-like appearance had left his hand in a great measure, and he was able to flex the fingers almost as well as ever, this being the first time he had done so since the fall down the stairs. From that time on, there was a steady improvement. I came to Mr. Parlin again in a week and had him sitting up and moving both arms. Soon after, he was walking about the room, and the fourth treatment I gave him was at the Worcester Post-Office Building, where I was then located. He had walked unaided from his home on Lancaster street, a distance of not less than three-quarters of a mile! He constantly improved in health, and at the time of this writing he has been at work nearly four years, as well and rugged a man as walks the streets. He weighs one hundred and seventy pounds and his rugged healthy appearance might well be envied by men of thirty years. His work consists of driving a big two-horse truck, and is strenuous enough to satisfy almost any men younger by many years.

Another rather singular case in the treatment of after effects of injuries was that of John J. Biu-ns, a freight conductor, employed by the Boston & Maine Railroad. Mr. Burns had his foot caught in the frog of a switch and badly crushed by a number of cars passing over it. The foot was badly misshapen after the wounds healed and the leg was also strained and distorted. This was a number of years previous to my knowing of him, but he suffered constantly from the effects of the accident. There was much pain in the limb at all times and it became of serious nature every time he took cold or any unusual strain or exertion occurred. This condition had persisted for fifteen years before I treated him. I considered the pain to be caused by restricted circulation in the muscles and the pressure which existed upon the nerves of the foot and leg. I treated the patient upon that supposition and immediately succeeded in increasing the flow of blood to the affected parts by the usual passes and suggestions. Since that time he has had no pain in the limb and its general condition has grown visibly better. It has been more than three years since I treated him and there has been no recurrence of the pain even under unfavorable circumstances.

CHAPTER IX

Heart Irregularities

FUNCTIONAL AND VALVULAR PROBLEMS –
FUNCTIONAL DIFFICULTIES EASILY RELIEVED –
TREATMENT – RAISED AS FROM THE DEAD – MRS. C'S
STRANGE RECOVERY – THE STRANGE CASE OF
THOMAS J HACKETT – RESCUED FROM TRANCE-LIKE
CONDITION AND SENSES RESTORED – HOW
INCURABLE CASES MAY BE RELIEVED AND LIFE
PROLONGED – HOW MISS H. LIVED FOUR YEARS
AFTER HER DEATH WAS DECREED

The heart is fortunately the most durable as well as the most vital organ of the body. There is no other organ that will perform its functions under such unfavorable circumstances as will the cardiac muscle. The diseases of the heart are generally spoken of in two classes, functional disturbances and valvular or organic diseases. A functional disturbance of the heart has some exterior source like acute indigestion or nervous depression. A valvular disease means the destruction or deterioration of some portion of the muscular tissue. It is probable that destroyed tissue in the heart muscle cannot be restored by any means any more than a new limb can grow to replace an amputated one; but even in the severest cases of valvular trouble, life and health can be prolonged by Natural Healing methods when no other curative agency can be of any avail whatever.

Functional heart troubles can be relieved by the skillful suggestionist quicker than by any other practitioner, since the causes of an irregular heart function can be reached successfully only through the subjective forces of life. Natural Healing removes the cause of functional heart trouble by stimulating the forces resident in the solar plexus and the inner nervous centers, and this is something that drug medication cannot hope to do. The treatment for heart difficulties must consist necessarily in the general stimulation of the subjective forces with the object of improving the general health and vitality. The general diagnosis of heart troubles is not usually difficult, as the symptoms of shortness of breath, especially after exertion, color of the lips, clutching or stabbing nature of pains in the left side, and, in severe cases, tendency to fainting, are ordinarily easily read signs. Many people, however, indeed it might be said the majority of people, have some form of heart irregularity and are never conscious of it during their entire lives because the organ has the remarkable power of "compensating," as it is called, for weakness in one part by enlarging the capacity of another to do more than its natural share of work. Generally the heart gives warning by easily recognized symptoms when it is being driven beyond its ability to respond.

One of the most remarkable cases I ever attended was one of severe functional heart trouble which threatened the patient's death. The case was notable, from my viewpoint, for two reasons : first, that I cured the patient when her death within the day was predicted by all attending her, save myself; and second, that she was entirely unconscious when I reached her bedside and objective suggestions could not reach her. I have explained my belief in the communication between subjective minds without objective intervention, and in this case which I am about to outline, it unquestionably took place, in my opinion. The patient was Mrs. C , the wife of a prominent manufacturer. She had suffered for a long time from a severe case of nervous exhaustion and her vitality seemed to be almost wholly exhausted. Her heart was affected and she finally became subject to periods of unconsciousness which were of very alarming nature. She suffered great pain and oppression in the base of the brain and spinal cord, and there were typical heart pains in the cardiac region. She of course had the best medical attendance, but she steadily grew worse until it finally became apparent that she could not survive many more attacks. At length she was taken with an alarming condition in the course of which she repeatedly relapsed into unconsciousness.

In the intervals of semi-consciousness, she repeatedly requested those about her to "Send for him." They could not at first make out who was intended, but finally some one asked if it was Mr. Gilson whom she meant, and before relapsing into unconsciousness she indicated that it was. It was the belief of those taking care of the patient that she could not live the day out, and immediately her husband decided to call me as a last resort. He did so, and when I arrived, Mrs. C was entirely unconscious and seemed to be breathing her last. I took her by the hand and strongly willed her to return to consciousness. I placed my right hand on the base of her brain and stimulated the centers vigorously. I exercised all the intention possible to make her rouse up and to relieve the overtaxed heart. In a few minutes I had the satisfaction of seeing her respond to the strong suggestions I was giving her mentally and she began to regain consciousness. In a little while she was fully conscious, and the manner in which she began to return to normal conditions was simply marvelous to those watching in the room. I gave her the strongest possible stimulation and suggestions to overcome the pain about the heart and the nervous depression.

In the course of a very few minutes she sat up in bed and wished to get up, but acting on my advice she did not do so for several hours. She then had a light lunch and from that time on began to gain rapidly. In less than forty-eight hours from my arrival at the house, the patient was out riding with her husband in their automobile. She continuously improved and has been in active health ever since. I have in my possession a very grateful letter from the lady's husband substantiating this account of this remarkable case in all essentials. It was of course a case of more or less spectacular nature, but to me it was of special interest because of the evidence it furnished to show that suggestions can be received subjectively or at least when the patient's objective consciousness is nonexistent.

An extremely strange case which illustrated the power of the mind to act subjectively, both in the giving and the receipt of suggestions, was that of Thomas J. Hackett, a young man about twenty years of age. Mr. Hackett was an armorer by trade and was employed in a well-known local factory. He had suffered for some time with ulcerated ears, and had been treated by specialists, but the trouble continued. Finally the pain became extremely severe, and lack of sleep, nervous strain and possibly some effect which the trouble may have had directly upon the brain, caused him to sink into a state resembling trance or partial catalepsy. He lost the senses of sight, hearing and taste, as well as the power of speech.

He was able to walk about and says he was conscious of what he was doing all the time, but he could not utter a word, hear a sound nor see anything except through a sort of dim haze. He remained in this extraordinary condition for a number of days. During that time he ate almost nothing. Finally he came to my office one morning, and a stranger looking individual I never saw. His face was set and mask-like, colorless and seemingly entirely without a spark of human intelligence or expression. He was led in and sat for some time in my waiting room without a movement that indicated his appreciation of anything outside himself. He seemed absolutely unconscious and heeded spoken words as little as would a granite block. When taken by the hand and guided, he would walk, sit down or stand up as he was directed to do, but otherwise he was not a sentient being as far as could be seen. A loud shout uttered suddenly behind him never caused him to wink an eyelash.

I believed on examining the patient that he was suffering from the effects of either great nervous shock or hypnosis, whether self-induced or not I could not tell. I saw he must be aroused from that state and I began work upon him. His ears were stopped up with cotton and his head wound with dressings, and these I removed at once. Then I began to stimulate his brain centers and exercise the most powerful possible intention to arouse him. I exercised forces calculated to counteract any hypnotic suggestions that might have been impressed upon him. I vibrated the ears strongly by placing my fingers in the orifices, and in short I tried all the expedients I was master of.

For some time he did not respond, but at last a faint flush began to come into his face and consciousness seemed to return or rather to manifest itself. Finally he began to make peculiar noises in his throat, and after more than half an hour of strenuous effort, he recovered his power of speech. In a little while longer I restored his hearing and finally his sight. He went home and ate voraciously and then went to sleep. On the following day he awoke in normal health, and soon returned to his work. All told, it was one of the most remarkable cases I ever met, for the young man stated to me afterward that he was conscious of his surroundings all the time, but unable to make any sound or to hear or see, except very dimly. He said it seemed like waking from a very hideous dream when I finally had succeeded in restoring him. Evidently his objective mind was not capable of receiving impressions through the senses, and the work was done by reaching him subjectively.

Another case which excited a considerable amount of attention at the time was that of Miss H, who was the victim of an organic heart trouble which it was evident to all must eventually terminate her life. She had been confined to her bed for weeks, and the opinion was given that it would be fatal for her even to stand upon her feet. Her trouble was a variety of heart lesion which very often produces sudden death, and it was the belief of her physicians that even slight physical exercise would result fatally. I was called into the case, and while I recognized that it was one in which life would be very brief comparatively, still I did not think the patient's time to die had arrived. I set myself to strengthen the heart action by the strongest suggestions I could bring to bear, and succeeded in gaining the patient's confidence in a gratifyingly short time. I then determined to attempt a radical experiment and I informed the young lady that she not only was not near her end, but was able to come out driving with me. She said she would do anything I thought wise, and I ordered her clothes brought, but owing to her long sickness she had no out-of-door clothing in readiness so I had her wrapped in the bed clothing and at my command she walked out to my carriage.

I kept her out in the air four hours that day and the next day she was up and walking about the house. I kept up the treatment steadfastly and the result was that the patient, whose death had been decreed as a matter of imminent certainty, lived four years longer, her life one of moderately active usefulness to her family and friends.

In the end she passed away quietly during my absence from the city, but the extension of her life for even four years was a thing of very gratifying nature both to her people and to me. It simply goes to show that the human mind when properly directed can preserve the body against the rapid progress of deterioration even when the process is too far advanced to hope for a permanent cure. In still another case I cooperated with a well-known physician of this city in the treatment of a case of internal cancer that was manifestly hopeless. I succeeded in prolonging the patient's life painlessly for more than two months longer than any medical prognosis could possibly hold out hopes of; and instead of dying in the agony such patients usually experience, this one passed away peacefully and seemingly with almost no suffering. I believe that such cases as these are as great triumphs in the art of relieving sufferings humanity as are the cases in which the disease is curable and the patient is restored to health. Every reader and student of this book who will devote himself to the earnest study and self-discipline that is necessary to develop his own subjective self can have the satisfaction and the pleasure of doing just these things and of relieving human pain and suffering wherever it is found.

CHAPTER X

Gastritis

OF THERAPEUTIC VALUE - VALUE OF SUGGESTIONS
NOT DEPENDENT UPON THEIR NATURE – DROPSY -
SYMPTOMS AND TREATMENT - DANGERS OF SALINE
CATHARTICS - INSPECTOR L'S

Gastritis is an ailment which has many apparent forms
and is closely allied to dyspepsia and nervous derangements of
the stomach function. The symptoms of dyspepsia and gastritis
are much alike in many respects; the same distress after eating
and the same formation of unpleasant gas in the stomach, the
eructation of food, etc., being noticeable. Nausea and
hiccoughing are generally marks of ailments of this nature, and
for the purposes of the operator, all forms of stomach disorder of
this sort may be grouped together and treated in similar manner.
The treatment by Natural Healing methods depends upon
suggestions, both mechanical and verbal, to overcome the
improper working of the stomach function. The flow of gastric
fluids is to be regulated by the stimulation of the abdominal
brain and the general stimulation of the brain and nerve centers
to be used in connection with strong suggestions against the
recurrence of the unpleasant symptoms after eating. Cases of
this nature yield more readily to suggestive methods than to
almost any other form of treatment; and when these methods are
used in conjunction with a proper regulation of the habits of
eating, sleep and exercise, cures are obtained in far the largest
percentage of the cases. A general health regimen that I have
found useful in many cases where the conditions were right for
its employment, is nothing more nor less than the much abused
and misunderstood "Kneip Cure," as it was called some years
ago.

THE LAW OF NATURAL HEALING

Like every other special form of mechanical suggestion, it has to be applied with judgment and under proper conditions. I have personally practiced it years before it ever became known publicly under the name of the German theorist, and I found it very beneficial. It consists in nothing more than walking bare-footed for twenty minutes or half an hour in the grass wet with the early morning dew. I have seen some really remarkable results obtained from this method. Naturally it cannot be undertaken by very weak people or those to whom a chill would be harmful, but a person of ordinary vitality can begin it in the late spring of the New England climate and persist in it daily till late in the fall with great benefit. It certainly requires no expensive apparatus and cannot do the least harm if begun under proper conditions. The patient simply rises early some fine late spring morning when the grass is wet with dew and walks about, minus his shoes and stockings, over some convenient lawn. Then on returning to the house, the feet should be bathed in warm water and dried carefully. This treatment can be carried out without danger into the late fall and I have known some robust persons who took so much pleasure in the treatment that they persisted in it long after the first light snow had fallen.

Contact with the earth in this manner certainly has a decided curative effect. With some patients the theory of the magnetists with reference to the cure will prove a beneficial suggestion. The exponents of magnetic theories claim that the negative or "back magnetism" with which the body becomes charged is taken out by contact of the bare feet with the earth, and the positive, or new and life-giving magnetism, is received from the atmosphere through the eyes at the same time. If such a belief or explanation will aid a patient in getting the best results, the thought can certainly do him no harm and may prove a very helpful suggestion. While no conscientious operator can of course countenance any wrongful falsehood or deceit that might lead to evil consequences, it is not always the best policy to combat strong beliefs of patients if they have a tendency to help their mental condition. An erroneous belief that helps a patient to exercise the curative forces within himself is surely better than no belief at all, or one that depresses and discourages him.

A suggestion is valuable not for what it is, but for what it does for the patient. All doing rests on faith in something and the object of the faith is immaterial, it is the existence of the faith that counts. So if a patient thinks he can be cured of rheumatism by a horse-chestnut carried in the pocket, I for one, would be glad to hunt up the horse-chestnut for him. It isn't the means but the end that makes a physician or a healer successful. To get the mind working in the right direction and to set free the mighty forces that exist within every human breast is the object of the Natural Healing practitioner, and the means, if within the boundaries of common right and probity, as indeed they must be, are not to be too critically analyzed. The physician knows that his bread-pill or his placebo would not be very efficacious if accompanied by a statement of its composition.

DROPSY is a disease condition marked by the accumulation of water in various tissues or in all the tissues of large areas of the body. The general form of dropsy shows the principal accumulation of water in the cellular tissue under the skin. Dropsy in which the water accumulates in the abdominal cavity is called ascites. Dropsy of the chest and of the brain are also common forms. The general treatment by ,the old school physicians has been to tap the patient and draw off the water in this manner. This can be done of course only when the location of the accumulation is such that no vital tissue will be pierced by the operation. Dropsy in the chest very frequently affects the heart action and finally kills the patient in that manner. Dropsy in the abdomen is marked by very great sense of pressure and swelling. The disease often makes its first appearance in swellings of the ankles. The patient is always pale and greatly run down in health and all the general functions are badly affected.

THE LAW OF NATURAL HEALING

The general treatment by Natural Healing methods is to stimulate the action of the kidneys as much as possible. The functions of elimination becoming deranged are the primary cause of dropsy, and the accumulations of water can only be safely removed by helping the kidneys to do more than a normal amount of work until the diseased condition is removed and the general health toned up to a point where the abnormal amounts of fluid will not be secreted in the tissues and cavities of the body. It has been found that use of saline cathartics in dropsy removes accumulations of water from the abdominal cavity, but that following their extended use, the amount of water is increased to a marked degree so that the net result of such treatment is a detriment to the patient. On the other hand the stimulation of the intestinal functions by Natural Healing methods shows no such reaction, and the kidneys and bowels can be made to work together to eliminate the abnormal fluid. I had one notable case of dropsy some years ago. Inspector L , of the Boston Police Department, came to me sufferering with a bad complication of asthma and dropsy. He had been tapped again and again, he told me, to relieve him of the great quantities of water which accumulated in the abdomen, accompanied with inflammation of the peritoneum.

At the time he first came to me, he was suffering greatly from asthma, but it was a period of comparative ease with him in respect to the dropsical trouble. I treated him according to the directions given heretofore for the cure of asthma. In two or three treatments he began to show a marked improvement. The process of elimination in the natural manner was set up and the asthma was very quickly conquered. The dropsy also began to abate very markedly and soon that also was gone. In a letter received from him more than a year after the course of treatment, he said that both troubles had disappeared entirely and he had not had any difficulty with either. His breathing was entirely easy and normal and he found no difficulty in walking or exercising to any normal extent.

CHAPTER XI

Some Notable Cases

DISEASES OF THE THROAT – HOW MRS. D.D.P WAS
CURED – SAVED FROM STARVATION – HOW ANDREW
J.M'S LIFE WAS SAVED MY NATURAL HEALING – ST.
VITUS' DANCE – GENERAL TREATMENT – MISS ALICE S.
RESCUED FROM CRITICAL CONDITION – MR. A'S SON
ANOTHER CASE

Very many in number and are of great variety, so much,
that the limits of a volume like this will not permit any extended
discussion of them. Such as are not of acute nature, like tonsilitis
in its acute form, laryngitis, diphtheria, etc., are to be treated in
the general manner with the purpose of allaying whatever
inflammation there may be, and stimulating the general functions
to remove the cause of the condition, which will in a very great
many instances be found to exist in improper nutrition and
elimination.

Some special cases of peculiar throat troubles I have
treated with success may be given as interesting illustrations of
the great variety of ailments the Natiu-al Healing operator is
likely to meet with in the course of a few years' practice. Mrs. D.
D. P, the wife of a former well-known Worcester citizen, had
suffered for three years with a muscular or nervous affection of
the throat which prevented her taking any food except in a liquid
form. The throat had a constant tendency to close up the passage
to the stomach, and mechanical means had to be resorted to in
order to allow the passage of food at all. Once a week the
attending physician was in the habit of stretching the throat with
instruments in order to keep the passage to the esophagus open
sufficiently to allow even liquid food to enter the stomach. She
was unable to sleep and she got hardly enough nutrition to keep

her alive.

I treated her in the general manner and made the usual passes over the throat, giving strong suggestions to relax the throat and allow the muscles to resume their natural position. Improvement was noted after the very first treatment. I attended her several times and within a few days after my first visit she was able to eat solid food. She gained twenty two pounds inside of six months from the beginning of my treatment, although when I commenced on her case, it was not thought she could ever rally her strength, she was emaciated to such an extent. This was a number of years ago and the patient is now as well as ever and has had no trouble whatever with either throat or general health since that time. Andrew J. M, of Worcester, was a man in advanced middle age who had worked all his life at the occupation of a painter. He had inhaled so much of the poison from the materials he worked with that he finally broke down completely and showed all the symptoms of paralysis. He was seemingly at death's door when I was called to see him. His whole side was useless and his throat was in such condition that he could not speak aloud, and only with the greatest difficulty could he take even small quantities of food. He had tried all the resources of ordinary medicine but made no material gain. His inability to eat was resulting in a process of slow starvation. He was not only terribly run down in bodily health, but his mind was so much depressed that it was pitiful to see him.

I went to see Mr. M and in a single treatment had him so he could speak and swallow. The treatment consisted solely of the usual methods of passes over the throat and affected limbs, strong intention on my part and firm suggestions which immediately took effect. The day following my visit, the patient was able to go to a neighboring town on a fishing trip. He steadily improved and his health was excellent, barring an organic heart trouble with which he had been a sufferer for years. This finally ended his life at the age of about sixty years, but he had no more difficulty, during the years between my treatment and his demise, from the trouble which it was declared would end his life immediately.

ST. VITUS' DANCE is one of the most distressing nervous ailments known. It is commonest in children, but occasionally settles into a chronic condition which lasts a lifetime. It is marked by involuntary and spasmodic movements of the muscles, twitching and jerking motions of the head, face, limbs and hands. The patient often finds difficulty in controlling the organs of speech, and inability to speak without stammering or stuttering when excited or surprised often occurs. In some cases the body of the patient is almost never still, the contortions and spasmodic movements being very painful to watch. It is believed to be entirely a nervous trouble, with its cause lying in obscure sources of malnutrition or other reasons for improper nervous action.

Its general treatment must necessarily be like that of other nervous troubles, special attention being paid to digestion, assimilation and elimination. The nerves need to be built up by a general systemic improvement, but the distressing symptoms can be cured in very short order by the proper use of Natural Healing methods. The patient and his friends will naturally look for relief from the outward symptoms which make the patient's life so miserable as the thing most to be desired, though really the treatment must go much deeper than that. The cases I have met with in the course of my practice have included some very severe ones, and I have found no difficulty in quelling the annoying nervous contortions almost at once, after which the process of renovation went on in its natural course without the knowledge of the patient. One of the most remarkable cases I have had in this connection was that of Miss Alice S, a young lady whose mother was a well-known professional nurse in Worcester. She had been sick with St. Vitus' dance for a long time and her case was complicated with other nervous disorders to such an extent that she was practically helpless. Her whole left side was useless and her tongue swelled to twice its normal size so that she could not utter a word in anything like a normal tone.

The best physicians in the city treated her, but they were unable to do her any good, and her mother was in despair about the child when she enlisted my aid in the case. I found the patient lying helpless in an invalid chair. I decided, on examination, that she would be easily amenable to suggestions. I gazed fixedly at her for a time and then ordered her to rise and walk, telling her in the most positive tone that she could do so. At first she demurred, but at a second command she rose and walked about the room. She had not been able for more than two months to raise her hand higher than her shoulder, and at my command she picked up a chair and lifted it above her head.

The spasmodic movements of her muscles began to disappear almost at once and in a very few treatments she was in practically a normal condition. Her improvement continued steadily and she has had no recurrence of it in four years' time. Although her sickness occurred at a critical period in a child's age, she has developed mentally and physically in the most gratifying manner, showing no ill effects whatever in after years. Another case of St. Vitus^ dance was exhibited by a young son of Mr. A , a prominent business man. He was learning the piano and it was thought that too close application to study produced the nodding and swaying motions of the head which made the poor child's life unhappy. In his case, I stimulated the various nerve centers and placing my hands on the back of the boy's neck, firmly suggested that he would have no more of the trouble. The difficulty grew less marked from that time, in the course of a very few treatments it had disappeared altogether and he was able to resume his musical studies almost at once.

CHAPTER XII

Bright's Disease

MAY BE CURED IN EARLY STAGES - RELIEF POSSIBLE
AT ALL TIMES - MARSHAL MARTEL'S REMARKABLE
CURE - OTHER CASES - DROP WRIST - LEAD POISONING
THE COMMON CAUSE – MR. A. H. A CURED BY A
SINGLE TREATMENT - OTHER EXAMPLES – GOITRE -
SOURCE OF INFECTION IN DIGESTIONAL FUNCTION -
MRS. JENNIE CURED OF SEVERE CASE OF GOITRE
JAUNDICE – TREATMENT

Brights' disease of the kidneys is supposed to be entirely incurable unless taken in the very earliest stages, and even then the medical authorities disagree upon the possibility of cure. It is characterized by the presence of albumen In the urine instead of sugar as in diabetes, but the products thus present are the result of actual destruction of the tissues themselves rather than a mere failure to perform their functions. In all probability the disease can be arrested in its early stages by Natural Healing methods in the majority of cases, but after a great deal of tissue is destroyed, it is not probable that Nature makes any provision for restoring it. I have no doubt, however, that the progress of the disease can be retarded in almost every case by means of suggestions, even if a cure cannot always be accomplished. One case that I have had seemed to indicate that the subjective forces can be aroused sufficiently to combat the disease even when it has progressed to some length.

Mr. Marshal Martel, a resident of Ayer, Mass., was the sufferer. He stated when I first saw him that he had been suffering with the disease for a long time. The amount of albumen present was very large and the treatment he had undergone had proved useless. Specialists he had consulted considered his case incurable. He was scarcely able to move about when I first treated him and was greatly wasted away. The symptoms of puffiness under the eyes, heart irregularity and emaciation of the body with dropsical tendency in the limbs were all to be observed.

I treated him for general systemic conditions together with local treatment over the kidneys and suggestions which would tend to increasing the general activity of the kidneys and bowels. The success of the treatment was marked. He began to improve almost at once and gained strength and weight in a notable degree. The general symptoms of the trouble disappeared in the course of a few weeks and the result of my half dozen or more treatments was a complete cure. He is apparently in normal health at this time.

Mr. C. E. S , of Nashua, N. H., was also a sufferer from inflammation of the kidneys. His urine displayed a great many foreign products and he often passed large quantities of blood with it. His strength was badly sapped by this condition and when I first treated him he was barely able to lean up against the wall as I did so. In a very short time the passing of blood ceased and the deposits in the water vanished, leaving it clear and normal. He gained strength rapidly and had no further disagreeable experience from the ailment, which was, in my opinion, a chronic inflammation of the entire urinary tract.

DROP WRIST, dropped instep, flat foot and a number of other kindred complaints are affections of the joints which are caused by the relaxation of the muscles and tendons through some cause which probably primarily works on the nerves. Drop wrist is a trouble very often experienced by painters, who absorb a great deal of lead into their systems. Flat-foot or dropped instep is often suffered by nurses and others who spend a great deal of time upon their feet, especially when wearing light foot-wear or slippers. A number of these cases have come to my attention and they have all yielded readily to suggestive methods. The nervous centers have to be stimulated and the subjective forces set to work, for there are no known medical expedients which will reach such cases, and mechanical supports in the cases affecting the feet are but a temporary relief. Braces and supports like plates in the shoes are frequently used in cases where the instep or ankles are affected. Drop wrist or "painters' disease," is a serious one because it wholly incapacitates the victim for his work. The hands hang useless from the wrists and flap about as though the joints were broken. No medicine that is known will relieve the trouble and the patient generally has to abandon his vocation completely. One or two cases of this kind have been included in my practice and have been cm*ed with gratifying ease.

Mr. A. H. A was a house painter who suffered a severe attack of drop-wrist after having worked years at his business and having gotten his system saturated with the lead poison. He could secure no relief and when he came to me his hand was entirely useless to him. I treated him but once and he immediately began to feel renewed strength in his wrists. The circulation was greatly improved and the blood was relieved of the poisonous matter by the natural process of elimination. The improvement was steady and the strength returned to the affected parts so quickly that the patient was able to resume work in a short time. Another young man, a Mr. S , suffered from dropwrist as the result of his work as a lead-burner or worker in that metal. He pursued a long course of drug medication before coming to me, but no strength returned to his hand. After a single treatment at my office he was able to use his hand with considerable freedom and secured a place where the work required was light. In a short time his wrist became strong and he experienced little if any difficulty with it thereafter. Another case in which the ankle joint was attacked was that of Mr. J. H, C, of Nashua, a clerk whose work required him to be on his feet a number of hours daily. For two years he suffered more or less pain and weakness in the ankle and finally he was about to submit to a surgical operation in the hope of a cure. He had worn a metal plate in his shoe for a long time to prevent the instep from falling flat with the rest of the foot. I treated him by vibrating the affected foot between my hands and immediately he could feel the circulation start and the foot tingled as though an electric current were passing through it. The pain subsided and within a very short time the strength had so far returned that he discarded the plate and has not since been troubled in the least.

GOITRE is a very common complaint in some localities, especially in damp regions. It is a swelling of the thyroid gland situated in the front of the neck. The name of the disease is derived from the symptom of protruding eyeballs which is commonly one of the first indications of the disease noticed. The gland swells to abnormal size and frequently presses upon the arteries and air passages so that feelings of suffocation are experienced. The disease is one of the digestive functions primarily and results from the filtration of the serous portion of the blood into the gland, which then becomes hypertrophied and often attains enormous size. Since it is a disease due to deranged digestive function, the general treatment should be vigorously resorted to. It should be recognized that the cure will require time, as the systemic change needed must be a gradual one. Local treatment and suggestions can be directed toward reducing the size of the swelling and obviating the unpleasant symptoms of pain and suffocation.

Mrs. Jennie S, of Fitchburg, Mass., had suffered two years with a goitre which finally assumed large proportions. It greatly weakened her by reason of the digestional disturbances which accompanied it, and she became greatly run down nervously as well as in flesh and strength. The case was pronounced to be one of incurable goitre. The swelling became so large that when she lay down she would have to raise her head with her hands in order to get up again. I was called into the case and found that it would be a long fight, but the patient was willing to follow directions faithfully. I commenced by treating the seat of the whole trouble, which I believed to be the intestinal tract. Local treatments dispelled the pain, but the general treatment was directed wholly toward securing the necessary systemic change.

In the course of three months the patient was completely cured. The swelling had disappeared entirely and the general physical condition was better than it had been for years. Digestion and nervous energy were alike completely renovated.

JAUNDICE is a condition accompanying almost all liver complaints and is. recognized from the yellow tinge imparted to the skin by the bile, which gets into the blood instead of being passed into the gall as it should be. All liver complaints can be treated after the general system, as outlined in the treatment of diabetes, except that the suggestions should be made to comport with the condition of the liver. In bilious troubles the suggestions are of course to prevent the passage of the bile into the blood and to regulate the general functions of the organ.

CHAPTER XIII

A Variety of Ills

FEVERS - HOW NATURAL HEALING CAN COPE WITH
THEM - DISEASES OF THE EYE – DEAFNESS - DISEASES
OF THE SKIN MR. GETCHELL CURED OF ACNE
WITHOUT THE USE OF DRUGS HAY FEVER – CATARRH -
TO BE COMBATED BY SYSTEMIC TREATMENT –
ANEMIA - ALCOHOLISM AND DRUG HABITS CURED BY
FRIGHT - LOCOMOTOR ATAXIA - A CASE WHERE
NATURAL HEALING BIDS FAIR TO CURE THE
INCURABLE CANCERS - ONLY RELIEF LIES IN
NATURAL HEALING – INSANITY - MISTAKES IN
TREATMENT - A SAD CASE – TUBERCULOSIS CURED -
MISS O FINDS NATURAL HEALING BETTER THAN
SANITARIUM – INSOMNIA - ITS CAUSES AND
TREATMENT - DANGER OF OPIATES

Fevers are conditions of the body recognized by
increased heat as shown by the thermometer, quickened
circulation changes in some of the tissues and disordered
secretions. Fevers are of many sorts and are acute conditions
where it is always necessary, in order to be on the safe side, to
employ drug medication. It has been explained why this is so.
Nature cannot rally the subjective forces quickly enough to
combat such crises without the help of internal medication. If the
subjective forces had been trained from infancy it is probable
that such a crisis as a fever would not occur, since the infection
would not be able to find a lodgment in a body so protected since
early childhood. Or if it did in an exceptional case secure
lodgment, the subjective forces could combat it easily. But where
the forces have been neglected all the lifetime, it is not
reasonable to expect they can be summoned in an hour to do
the work of years. The Natural Healing operator, however, can

be of the greatest help in such crises even during the acute state and it is well known that very often a feverish temperature can be lowered by properly administered suggestion as easily as by a dose of some febrifuge. The Natural Healer and the physician can work together in such cases with great benefit, if they will, and directly the acute condition has passed, the operator can hasten convalescence in a marked degree. Suggestions can always be found useful in all circumstances if they are skillfully applied.

DISEASES OF THE EYE are very numerous and often are best treated by the oculist, especially where they are of such nature as can be reached by the use of glasses. Where they are of nervous origin, affecting the optic nerve and the visual centers, general systemic treatment together with local stimulation is the ordinary course of treatment. Water prepared as directed in a previous chapter by vibrating between the hands often offers a good means of suggestion. It can frequently be used as a wash with good effect.

Toning up the nervous energy often is all that is required to cure visual deficiencies. One case I had was that of an old lady who was nearly blind. She was brought to me to be treated for rheumatism which I succeeded in helping materially. To the great surprise of herself and her friends, her eyesight, which was thought to be an incurable factor in her case, was very much benefited and she could see with considerable ease by the time she completed her course of treatment.

DEAFNESS is the result of a number of causes. Often it follows other sicknesses like fevers, rheumatism, or catarrh. It is sometimes caused by the total demolition of the eardrum, or tympanum, either through disease or from accidents, loud explosions, etc. In such cases there is no cure, any more than there is for an amputated leg. When, however, the deafness is caused by inflammation of the membranes, as it often is, general systemic treatment with local vibrations and appropriate suggestions will effect a cure. The congestion in the tissues can be relieved and the circulation stimulated, which will restore the hearing in due course of time.

DISEASES OF THE SKIN are of many kinds and in general imply a disordered condition of the blood. They can best be approached through a course of treatment calculated to eliminate the impurities in the system and thus relieve the blood of the elements which produce the unsightly skin conditions.

I once cured a well known local merchant, Mr. I. G. G, of a red rash or acne of long standing, by a course of three treatments calculated to quicken the circulation and purify the blood. The acne disappeared in the course of a very few days and although during the time he had suffered from it, which was for more than four years, it was very unsightly and annoying, his face became smooth and the skin clear after the treatment. He has suffered no return of the trouble in the course of the several years which have elapsed since I attended him.

HAY FEVER is a common and troublesome ailment in New England. It exhibits many of the indications of asthma, but is not of the same nature. There is inflammation and irritation in the membranes of the nasal and throat passages as well as in the head. Some think it caused by the pollen of grasses and plants floating in the air, but it is probably of nervous origin, for if it were not, a change of climate would always cure it, which does not happen. The treatment is substantially the same as for asthma or any other condition in which the nervous system is deranged by the inaction of the functions of nutrition and elimination.

CATARRH is a term used to indicate certain inflammation of the mucous membrane. It occurs in many portions of the body and is especially common in the nasal and bronchial regions. It occurs in mild form in a great many people, some of whom suffer almost no perceptible inconvenience from it. In others it is very severe and wherever present is a factor detrimental to health because it produces a condition of systemic poisoning by reason of the discharges from the affected membranes. Catarrh may wholly destroy the membranes and produce the most fatal conditions of tuberculosis or it may exist in mild form during a patient's whole lifetime. It should be combated by general treatment for the digestion and the nervous system, the effort being directed toward eliminating the systemic poison. No medicines will do this and there is no power known save the concentrated force of the subjective mind that will eradicate catarrhal conditions.

Applications like sprays and inhalants are but local in their effects and the basic root of the trouble cannot be got at from without inward- it has to be an attack upon the enemy from within to drive him out. Catarrh can be cured by Natural Healing methods and by no other as far as is known, but it is necessary for patient and operator alike to devote their best and most intelligent efforts to the work and even then the results must come slowly as the general systemic change takes place.

ANEMIA is a deteriorated condition of the blood arising from impaired circulation. An observance of general rules of hygiene, outdoor air and exercise and generous diet of blood-making constituents will supplement the general treatment in effective manner. The degeneration of the blood is caused by a decrease in the normal number of red corpuscles and the suggestions given should be aimed toward stimulating the functions that control the making of new blood. Overwork is the cause of most anemic conditions, and the causes responsible for the condition should of course be looked into and corrected before the treatment is entered into.

ALCOHOLISM AND DRUG HABITS. In no portion of the Natural Healing operator's practice is there more opportunity for helping the weak and suffering members of humanity than in the treatment of habits which are beyond the control of the sufferers and fatal to their physical and spiritual welfare unless checked. Despite the existence of many institutions for the cure of liquor and drug habits, there is no medical treatment known that offers a certain cure. Suggestion alone can cure the victims of these habits permanently. In several cases, in which connection it is obvious that names cannot be used, I have succeeded in a very few treatments in utterly destroying the taste for injurious substances which the patients had not been able to control for years.

In one case a manufacturer in another New England city had long been a heavy drinker. He found its evil effects on his business were marked and he earnestly desired to abstain from the use of whiskey, which was his ordinary form of indulgence. I treated him several times, giving him strong suggestions against his ability to keep whiskey on his stomach. He was utterly unable to retain liquor after that time and in a short while was able to control the habit completely. Another case was that of a man who had been a confirmed drinker for years. He had descended about as low as it was possible for him to do when his employers asked me to see if I could do anything for him. He had suffered a slight shock of paralysis as the result of his habits and I found him in a, pitiable condition indeed. I treated him for his affected limb and when I had gotten him so he could walk about with much more ease than before, I saw I had gained his confidence. Then I suddenly turned upon him with a glare and a look of the utmost determination and told him dramatically that if he ever drank another drop of liquor, he would fall dead that instant!

The poor man looked as though he would drop at that, but he promised faithfully that he would not drink again and strangely enough the impression made upon him was so strong by that single suggestion that he never did touch liquor again. He could not be tempted to do so, and it was evident that he was utterly convinced that his end would occur if he broke the prohibition I had laid upon him! Such methods of course are not fair examples nor are they to be used indiscriminately, but they happened to fit the circumstances in this case to perfection!

LOCOMOTOR ATAXIA is one of the most dreaded of all nervous diseases and is still regarded by many medical practitioners as incurable. It may be so after the destruction of certain tissues has taken place. The cause of the disease lies in the hardening and indurating of the lower portion of the spinal column, causing the motor nerves to be pressed upon and their functions deranged. The patient cannot control the action of the lower limbs, stumbles and falls when attempting to walk and as the disease progresses loses almost wholly the control of the motor nerves. As the difficulty proceeds along the course of the spinal column, the condition grows worse till finally the patient becomes wholly a cripple, physically and mentally. If the disease is taken before the nervous ganglia are destroyed, it can be cm- ed by general treatment as indicated for all deranged nervous and other functions. The most favorable hygienic conditions of course have to be observed and the faithful compliance of the patient with all the necessities of the treatment is perhaps more essential in ataxia than in any other disease. Like nervous prostration, it can be conquered only by the fully concentrated forces of the mind.

A recent case of locomotor ataxia m my practice was one where the ailment had existed for some time, but the symptoms did not warrant the belief that nervous tissue of vital nature had been destroyed. The patient was unable to walk with any certainty and could do almost no work. I began with a course of general treatments and finding him easily amenable to suggestion I succeeded in directing his mind to his own help in a short time. The case is at this time progressing slowly, but from inability to do any work of much account, the patient is now able to work full time in a factory where his occupation is running a stamping press actuated by a push of his foot. Needless to say he could not have done any such work as this when the treatment began.

CANCER is one of the most dreaded of all diseases and since it is due to bacilli or germs which permeate the whole system, few operations by which the cancer is removed surgically result in permanent cure. I have no doubt that cancer can be cured by the subjective forces of the human mind if it can be cured at all, but I doubt if many individuals exist in whom it is possible to summon the forces quickly and strongly enough to effect a cure. Cancer is today practically an incurable disease, especially after the germs have spread from the original source of infection to the other tissues of the body. Natural Healing methods certainly offer the only real hope a cancer victim today has. There can be no doubt the power is within every man which can heal all diseases, but how often it can be developed in time to fight this most dangerous of diseases is problematical. Always, however, methods of suggestion can be used to stay the progress of the disease and to lessen the pain which all its victims suffer. If taken in its early stages, I am confident that many cases of the disease can be cured by the skillful Healer.

INSANITY is of very many forms, and except where there are irreparable lesions in the brain tissue, all should be cm-able. It is evident that drug medication in such diseases is futile. Suggestion alone can restore mental balance. The Natural Healing operator is not likely to have a great many cases of brain disease in the course of practice because of the public regulation of such cases, but still I have met with some in the course of my work. One case in particular was that of a young man who was a private patient in one of the state institutions. He was brought by permission of the authorities to be treated by me and as he was suffering from acute violent mania, it took several men to control him by main force. I treated him for a few minutes and inside of a quarter of an hour after my arrival at the house where he was staying, he was docile as a child. He would obey me readily and seemed actually to be entirely rational. He steadily improved during the few days I had opportunity to treat him, but owing to the opposition of relatives, he was taken back to the institution, relapsed amid the scenes of horror prevalent there and afterwards died. I have no doubt that a great many cases of insanity could be cured by separation from other insane patients and treatment by suggestive methods.

TUBERCULOSIS or consumption is probably the most widespread and most dreaded of all diseases. It is commonest as tuberculosis of the lungs, though any of the tissues of the body may be attacked by it. The disease called lupus, or "The wolf," common in some European countries, is tuberculosis of the skin. The commonly noted symptoms are emaciation, loss of strength, hectic flush, hollow coughing, hemorrhages from the lungs, daily periods of fever. Consumption is always complicated or accompanied by digestive irregularities and general functional disturbance. Treatment tending toward keeping up the general strength and regulating the functions of elimination, in combination with nourishing diet and complete out-of-door life in a dry atmosphere has proved itself the best method of procedure.

I had one case of tuberculosis of the lungs, who had been a patient for some time in a sanitarium for the cure of tuberculosis. She left the institution after a course of treatment and it was said that her lungs were still affected and that she could not be entirely cured. She came to me and after a few weeks of treatment according to the general method laid down, her health was very notably improved. An examination of her lungs by the sanitarium authorities shortly after showed that all tubercular symptoms had disappeared and she has since enjoyed perfect health. I am convinced that methods of suggestion will hasten convalescence from tubercular affections very materially.

THE LAW OF NATURAL HEALING

In short, there is no human ill of any nature, in my belief, which cannot be minimized in its effects, if not completely cured, by the right use of the subjective power which is the heritage of every human being.

INSOMNIA, or sleeplessness is a condition that accompanies a great many nervous disorders and is very frequently a most serious phase of their progress. If not checked, mental and physical wreck is sure to result, for sleep is quite as essential to the human organism as food, perhaps even more so. The basic treatment for insomnia will of course be that given for the nervous condition which produces it, but the local treatment will include the strongest possible suggestions to aid the patient in overcoming the inability to sink into repose. Victims of insomnia frequently become so badly affected that they get but one or two hours' sleep a night and occasionally very serious cases get no sleep at all for several nights. Such cases are extremely dangerous and it is known that no human being can go an entire week without sleep and live, while sanity may be destroyed by even shorter periods of wakefulness.

The condition called sleep is regarded scientifically as being caused by a natural withdrawal of the blood from the brain tissues in a manner analogous to the condition that pertains when unconsciousness from syncope occurs, except that, being a natural function, it has no ill, but rather beneficial effects upon the general organism. In theory at least, therefore, sleep can be induced mechanically by the withdrawal of blood from the brain tissues and the usual expedients adopted are warm baths for the feet, cold plunges or packs for the entire body, ice upon the head, or any similar expedient that will withdraw the blood from the brain. Some nervous specialists treat insomnia patients with strong mustard or other drawing plasters upon the bottoms of the feet on going to bed.

The principle upon which all opiates act is the forcing of

blood from the brain, but the use of opiates in insomnia is a fatal proceeding, for the reaction ensuing upon the use of such drugs necessitates larger and larger doses and their effects after long continuance of use are too well known to require comment. The only safe and efficacious means for the relief of insomnia is found m. the use of Natural Healing methods, while its cure can only lie in the eradication of the nervous conditions underlying it. It is obvious that the skillful use of suggestion is the only means known to hasten Nature's process of repairing the waste of nervous tissue that produces neurasthenic conditions.

The treatment for insomnia should be given preferably just before the patient retires. The general treatment for the nervous trouble can of course be given at any time, but the special treatment is best given just before sleep is to be induced. The treatment should consist of passes down the sides of the head, neck and body accompanied by the statement that the blood is to follow the course of the operator's hands, relieving the brain tissues and carrying away the excess of blood from the arterial to the venous system. Then the suggestions of sleep can be given firmly and impressively, and if the operator takes the patient's hand in his, gazes fixedly into his eyes and passes his hand lightly over the sufferer's eyes and brow, he will very often have the satisfaction of seeing the sick man drop gently off to sleep in a most natural and refreshing manner.

If it is not desirable to use this method or it does not at once prove effective, a glass of water prepared in the prescribed manner and administered with the suggestion that it will have immediate opiate effect, will generally act almost instantly. All troubles of this nature are to be recognized as purely nervous in origin and treated accordingly. Local treatment is only for relief-the root of the matter must be gotten at and the patient must understand that a restoration of the nervous vitality is a process requiring time and faithful application.

CHAPTER XIV

Breathing the Best Hygienic Precaution

THE VITAL NEED OF OXYGEN IN ALL THE TISSUES -
HOW TO BREATHE – EXERCISES - AN ORIGINAL
METHOD - A HYGIENIC MEASURE WITH A REAL
PSYCHIC JUSTIFICATION - HOW FAR TO CARRY ANY
EXERCISE

Among all the hygienic precautions and exercises that can be prescribed, the most important are those which have to do with breathing. The oxygen of the air is the vital fluid of physical life and it is absolutely essential to the processes which go on within the physical being and constitute the condition which is called living. A very large percentage of all human ailments might be traced at least indirectly to a failure to secure enough oxygen to supply bodily needs. The function of oxygen is simply to afford the possibility of combustion. The human body works exactly as does the fire in a furnace under a boiler. It takes certain carboniferous elements and by the process of combustion, which is only the union of such elements with oxygen at a certain necessary temperature, converts them into other forms which are required to produce heat or force or energy. The elements which enter the body cannot be absorbed or used by it unless they undergo this process of oxidation, and the portions of the fuel products not required by the body can only be eliminated from it by further process of oxidation.

Therefore if a person does not get sufficient pure air containing the required proportion of oxygen, his body not only does not get the good from the food elements which enter it, but fails to eliminate the baser elements which are not useful but positively harmful to it. A man can live without food for many days and without water for many hours, but he cannot live even a very few minutes without air. The importance of breathing exercises can never be sufficiently emphasized. The majority of persons breathe with only a small portion of their lungs. The born idiot breathes only with the extreme top of his. The coward betrays himself in a narrow chest and a breathing habit that fills only the upper half or less of his natural air capacity. Smallness of character and mind is almost always shown by improper breathing.

The American Indians declared that only the boaster and the coward breathed through their mouths- men breathe through their nostrils. Full, deep breathing is the natural concomitant of calm, well-ordered thinking and a clean, well disposed order of life. Getting enough air into the lungs at every breath is an essential to physical health and therefore to the mental health and spiritual well-being. It is well to breathe deeply and fully no matter how it is done, but there are certain right ways of breathing as well as of doing everything else in life and their mastery is a factor of well-being and success to every student and reader of this volume. A few general exercises for deep breathing may be given, though these can be found in almost any text-book of hygiene or athletic manual. All breathing exercises should be taken in the open air with the lips tightly closed, but not compressed in a self-conscious or uncomfortable manner. If for any reason, the patient cannot go out of doors in all weathers, the breathing exercises should be taken before an open window, avoiding a draught.

Exercises should not be taken upon a full stomach, though moderate breathing exercises will do no harm even then. 1st Exercise,- Stand erect, heels together, spine straight, head high, but not thrown back unnaturally, eyes looking on a level, hands hanging by the sides naturally. Place the hands on the waist in such manner that the middle fingers meet in front, the thumbs pointing backward. Inhale slowly through the nostrils, sending the air down deep so that it seems to force the middle fingers apart. Hold the air for a second or two, then expel slowly through the nose til there is a feeling of relaxation at the waist. Repeat this several times at the first trial.

2nd Exercise.- Place the hands at the sides of the waist and breathe as before, gently pressing on the ribs as the exhalation takes place.

3rd Exercise.- Place the hands at the small of the back and repeat as before, without pressing the waist at all during the exercise. Always aim to throw the breath low down in the chest, but do not strain the lungs nor produce a marked feeling of exhaustion, as that is necessary. The object should be to make the lungs feel as though they themselves and not the muscles, were doing the breathing. That is, make the act of inhalation seem like one of the will and not of pure muscular action.

4th Exercise.- Stand in the first position with hands at the sides and draw in a slow deep breath while you count eight. Hold the breath while you count eight; then count eight while exhaling. Repeat a number of times. The exercises at first should only occupy two or three minutes, especially in the case of persons who are not strong or who have not been accustomed to exercises of the sort and whose breathing is naturally deficient. The time can be lengthened rapidly each day, however, and within a few weeks, fifteen minutes in the morning before breakfast, and the same at night before retiring, with whatever other periods are convenient during the day, will not be too much. The fourth exercise can be taken to good advantage while walking at a moderate gait in the open air. Walking is one of the best, of exercises when accompanied by proper breathing, but it. should always be at a steady, calm, deliberate gait. Hurried, nervous walking does more harm than good.

Aside from these directions for ordinary breathing, there is a method but little known, and indeed I do not know that it has ever before been published, which has not only physical but real mental value to recommend it. This exercise not only answers all the purposes of a good physical breathing exercise, but it also promotes subjective activity and directs, the hidden forces to the stimulation of the involuntary functions. Its beneficial effects in disciplining the mental forces and strengthening them are, to my own knowledge, very great. The procedure should be as follows: Seat yourself alone in a quiet room where there will be no chance of disturbance. Separate the mind as much as possible from surrounding material conditions and strive to render it passive. The body should be disposed in an easy sitting position, but in such manner that the chest will not be cramped. Then when a state of suitable mental and physical repose and passivity has been attained, the exercise may be commenced.

Close the right nostril with the right forefinger laid upon the side of the nose. Close the eyes and breathe deeply and slowly through the left nostril, letting the inhalation last while five is counted in slow cadence. Send the breath deep into the chest and when this method of breathing through the left nostril is used, a very different sensation from that of breathing through both nostrils is experienced.

You will feel a current of cold air go down into the chest and around the region of the heart. Force the breath deeper and deeper till it seems to go far down into the abdomen and proceeds across the front of the body. Hold the breath in this manner till five can be counted; then exhale through the right nostril while five is being counted. At the conclusion of the period of holding the breath, the forefinger should be lifted from the right nostril and the middle finger laid upon the left nostril, closing it and leaving the right free for exhalation. This process should be repeated two or three minutes the first day and increasing periods later.

Auto-suggestions given during the inhalation periods are

119

found to have the strongest possible effect and this method of breathing and self-treatment has not only been of much use to me, but has cured many patients of various diseases.

All breathing exercises as well as all physical exercises of all natures should not be carried to the point of marked fatigue. It has often been erroneously supposed that muscular exercise ought to be persisted in until extreme fatigue is felt, in order to be useful in developing the body. That is not the case, for fatigue is a sign of the destruction of tissue, not of its upbuilding.

Nature provides an infallible guide to determine the point at which exertion of all sorts should stop. As long as it is possible to breathe through the nose it is generally safe to say that exercise is not being carried beyond the safety point of strain upon the heart and lungs and the other vital tissues. As soon as it is necessary to open the mouth in order to breathe, the danger point is being passed and exercise should be abated till a period of rest has elapsed.

CHAPTER XV

Some Suggestive Expedients

THE HOT AND COLD BREATH – IDEAL SUGGESTION –
PROFESSOR WOOD'S THEORY - NATURAL HEALING
CAN DEVELOP THE SPIRIT AS WELL AS CURE THE
BODY - HIGHEST IDEALISM AS WELL AS MATERIAL
SUCCESS WITHIN THE NATURAL HEALER'S PROVINCE

The breath can be used as a powerful factor in giving healing suggestions in certain kinds of cases, and sometimes the student will find valuable help in treating some of his patients in a simple expedient that I have discovered and used myself. It is the use of hot and cold breath, which despite the Aesopan fable, can be blown from the same mouth to good purpose sometimes! A moment's experiment will show the student that if he breathe upon his hand or upon that of another, with the mouth held close to it and the lips and teeth wide apart, the resulting sensation will be of marked heat. On the contrary if the lips are held in the position of whistling and the breath blown gently through them, the hand held at a distance of an inch or two will feel a pleasant cooling sensation. In cases of inflammation, a cool breath blown upon the affected part will prove grateful in sensation and, if accompanied by appropriate suggestions, will often relieve and dispel the condition. In cases of congestion, on the other hand, such as occur in facial neuralgia, etc., place a clean handkerchief on the patient's flesh and blow the hot breath through it and the sensation of heating will prove a good vehicle for potent suggestions of curative nature.

In some cases the very exposition of the ability to blow hot and cold will arrest the patient^s attention and secure his confidence to his own great good. The means used to convey suggestions may often seem petty and almost amusing to the educated operator, but it is not the means of imparting suggestions, but the mighty curative power of the forces affected by them that counts. Prof. Wood employs the suggestive theory in a somewhat novel manner in the endeavor to develop the spiritual side of man's being. He devotes his efforts to the inculcation of the highest moral idealism, considering that the spiritual development is the one real object of worthy endeavor. He aims at the highest things first, believing that the physical body will be healed of itself when the divine heritage of which he speaks has been attained, that is, the birth of the spiritual consciousness and the freedom of man from the Dominion of sin and selfishness.

He adopts what he terms "Ideal Suggestions," which are suitable auto-suggestions, and these he strives to impart by what he calls "Mental photography," which is the repetition of suggestions while in a state of mental and physical passivity, until they have been impressed on the subjective mind through objective repetition backed by the direction of the will. His system consists in having the suggestions printed on cards in large letters. Each suggestion is accompanied by a dissertation upon which the student is required to meditate before the process of repetition is begun. Then the card with the appropriate suggestion is placed in easy view while the state of passivity is induced.

The student fixes his eyes upon the card, banishing all other impressions save the form and meaning of the suggestion in question. His concentration upon the card and its printed sentence is supposed to imprint or photograph its likeness upon the objective mentality whence it is transferred in the manner of all suggestions to the subjective mind. These suggestions, as outlined by Prof. Wood, are of a nature particularly to appeal to people of a religious bent, but of course any others could be substituted for his series. As a mechanical aid to auto-suggestion, many patients might find this plan very efficacious. The idea of mental photography, in this connection, is in itself an ingenious suggestion. Thus far, the whole aim of this work has been to show how the powers of the mind can be directed toward the improvement of physical conditions.

Physical health is, from one point of view, the most important factor m human life. In very few cases indeed is it possible for a human intellect, spirit or soul, let it be called what one will, to attain its highest development in a diseased physical tenement. The body and the mind are connected in so close and mysterious a fellowship that the impoverished body, assailed by unnatural conditions, hampers and drags down the higher attributes of the spirit. The noblest work, the highest thinking, cannot be done by a mind chained to a diseased and suffering body. So that the search for physical health as a means to higher mental growth, is the most worthy pursuit a man can follow. It has been attempted to show, with what success the reader will determine, that the subjective forces of the human mind offer the best and surest means of securing perfect physical conditions, because in them is the control of those conditions and nowhere else is such control lodged. The desire, backed by the will, to be strong and well physically, is all that man needs to attain a perfect physical condition. This being so, how much wider and nobler a field is there open to every one in the development of the mind and soul through the application of the suggestive theory to man's latent potentialities.

Prof. Henry Wood says in his admirable book on this subject: "The purpose of ideal suggestion is far broader and higher than the mitigation and healing of physical ailments, however desirable that may be. Such is but an incidental part of its work, and the same is true of mental healing as that term is ordinarily employed. The grand mission of these great principles is the development of the spiritual ego; to roll away the stone from the door of the sepulcher of the lower self; to bring to birth the spiritual consciousness; to free man from the dominion of sin and selfishness, and to enthrone the real divine self,- God's image,- and put him in possession of his divine heritage." No object of scientific investigation offers such wide possibilities, since none other comes so near to the root of things as does research into the workings of the subjective forces. There is no human activity of any nature in which the subjective entity of mankind does not exercise, even though unconsciously, a dominant influence. From the correcting of the most insignificant physical ill to the realization of the highest spiritual idealism, the power that does is within man's own being.

Whether a man seek physical health, material prosperity or the grandest ideals of spiritual altruism, his ability to attain is measured in direct proportion to his subjective development. So that the student of subjective phenomena does not find himself limited merely to the acquirement of knowledge that "Ideal Suggestion through Mental Photography." Henry Wood cures the bodies of others, but he sees opened to him the grandest truths of ethical and moral philosophy which he can apply in securing for himself and others enlarged material, mental and spiritual growth. Not alone perfect physique but increased material well-being, broadened personal influence and even character itself result from the wise training and directing of our Natural forces. It cannot be doubted that men who are "successful," in the ordinary terms of expression, are those who, by their development of what is known as personality or personal magnetism, are able to sway their fellow men to their own ends. This development is probably within the reach of all to a greater or less extent, and so long as its use is within the boundaries of what is known and recognized to be right and just, it is a perfectly legitimate and proper use of a great Natural force.

But no matter how honestly personal influence is used, it does not realize the highest ideals when it is employed solely for personal advancement and aggrandizement. Aside from the common object of physical improvement and on the other extreme, the ideal development of spiritual growth, there is a domain of practical everyday life in which the value of psychic development cannot be overestimated. The grand object of all human life is success, that is, the attainment of some specific goal toward which ambition points. The material manifestation of success is almost always money, position, influence. But whether these purely material manifestations or the better ones of artistic or ideal attainment are what spell success in any individual case, the end can only be gained by the development of the subjective powers. Observe any man who has "arrived," who has made his place, attained his goal, at least in a worldly sense. Invariably he will be found to possess certain qualities-those qualities which in the summation are called "personality", "personal magnetism" etc. He will be found to have either the ability to influence men to his will merely by the intangible force that surrounds his words and actions, or he will be found to have the ability to concentrate all his energies upon some one object and to pursue it through thick and thin to his end. He will have indomitable will and unflagging energy. One or all of these qualities will be found in every man who has succeeded, whether it be at money-getting, man-leading or picture-painting. These qualities are not natural gifts to one man more than to another. They are the natural heritage of all men, but they are developed either consciously or unconsciously in very different degrees. In the light of investigations into subjective phenomena, we know that health is teachable. Success is teachable also. What makes up the summation of life? Actions. What, are actions but the crystallization of thoughts into a form which is tangible to the physical senses? Thoughts are things. Thought is a wave motion in the ether, differing only from the vibrations that produce light, heat and electricity in the same way that a maple differs from an elm. Both are trees, but they differ in physical characteristics. Personal magnetism is the result of concentration of thought upon definite, appropriate lines and the development of the power to detect thought into definite, effective channels.

CHAPTER XVI

Teachability of Success

ADDUCTIVE POWER OF THOUGHT - "I CAN" AND
SUCCESS CAN BE TAUGHT – CONCENTRATION THE
FIRST REQUIREMENT – PRACTICAL DIRECTIONS – A
STORY TO ILLUSTRATE THE POINT

Thoughts seem to have the power of attracting their like. The mental atmosphere of one oppressed by fear or habitually thinking fear thoughts, is filled with fear to the exclusion of all other impulses or emotions. Fear breeds fear and so does every other class of thought attract and multiply itself from the great unseen reservoirs of thought vibration which surround us. The only difference between success and failure in life is the difference between a positive and a negative mode of thinking. The positive thinker thinks, "I can and I will"; and the negative thinker says to himself "I can."

All thought seems to possess this adductive power, the ability to draw to itself other thoughts of like kind. The man who thinks thoughts of failure attracts to himself all the thoughts of failure in his vicinity and he fails because his subjective mind which governs all his involuntary actions, which subconsciously registers all the experiences of life, has nothing but directions of failure to work upon. The pessimist and the man who looks for evil, auto-suggests himself into the very circumstances he forecasts. The objective mind is the active half of the mentality. It perceives, reasons, considers, accepts, rejects. The subjective mind is the passive element. It believes everything the objective mind sends to it through the will. It acts on every impulse it receives unless restrained by a stronger opposite one. The man whose objective mind is constantly on guard to prevent the subjective mind from getting anything but the kind of impressions that tend to success is the man who believes in himself- that is in the divine power that is within himself, the ego. He is the man who succeeds, while he who constantly believes in failure and misfortune gives the passive element of his mind the very kind of directions that hasten him on to ruin.

While there is no doubt about the teachability of success, it is not always the easiest thing to break away from old thought habits and to set the objective mind at work guarding the subjective or passive function from bad impressions.

Concentration is the keynote of subjective control. Learn to do things one at a time and with all the might. No one who has not tried knows what a difficult thing it is to control the attention. Concentration upon one definite thing to the utter exclusion of everything else is one of the hardest possible feats, but it is the secret of successful endeavor in every activity of life. A few practical directions for securing the ability to concentrate may be given. A great many people waste half their energy in involuntary movements of the muscles and nerves, some of which become so habitual that they are unconsciously done. Useless, nervous motions, like swinging the feet when sitting down, rocking continuously, playing with small objects, like pencils, watch-chains and guards, swaying movements, drumming with the fingers and all similar manifestations of nervous temperament are objectionable because they distract the attention from more important things. They also use up nervous energy that might better be devoted to more useful ends.

Learn to sit quietly, easily, avoiding tense muscles when they are not in use. It is easy to form such a habit of carrying the body as it is to form the useless habits just spoken of and a little practice and attention will change the old habits into the new one in a little while. Then when these involuntary nervous affairs have been corrected, begin to train the voluntary attention and see how difficult a thing it is to master. The attention is a most unruly servant and tends to wander in all sorts of paths unless kept strictly to the business at hand. The power to concentrate the attention can only be secured by practice.

Some simple expedients may be adopted that will greatly help in this connection. One is to take an easy sitting position in a place where there will be no disturbance and hold a common lead pencil or some other uninteresting object in the hand. Gaze firmly upon it and think of nothing but it. Fix the attention upon it as though there was nothing else in the world but you and it. Consider it in every possible light, as to shape, size, color, length, use, origin, process of manufacture, value, sale, and in every other connection that ingenuity can suggest. But don't let the thoughts wander from the pencil itself into any of the side channels these reflections will open. When you have mastered the ability to think hard, not merely gaze idly, upon a simple object of this sort, you will find that you have secured a very valuable training and one that will help you immeasurably in all thought afterward. An old story is told of a lawyer who wished to take a youth into his office in the old days when lawyers were made in that way, that is, by study in the offices of their seniors. He let his intention be known and, as he was a man of much repute, the applicants were many. He made his choice from the large number of boys by a novel method which determined to his satisfaction that the successful one would exhibit the proper legal turn of mind.

He took each applicant separately and told him a long story which began with the incident of a squirrel running down a tree and into a hole in the side of a barn. From this point the story branched out in a multitude of detail and contained some startling incidents, like the breaking loose of the cattle in the barn, the burning of the structure, the killing of the owner by a fall from the fire ladder and other features of surprising nature, all told in the most graphic manner. At the conclusion of the tale he asked each listener for some comment on it. One questioned about the origin of the fire, another about the worth of the structure, another about the number of cattle lost, and so on, and each was rejected. At last one little freckled-faced fellow listened attentively all the way through and then as he sat silent at the end, the lawyer encouraged him to ask a question. "Isn't there anything else you'd like to know about it?" he asked. "Well," said the boy finally, "I'd like to know what became of that squirrel!", "You're the one," said the lawyer in delight, "You're engaged!"

The boy was the only one of the lot that had been able to grasp a fact, concentrate upon it and stick to it, despite all the mist of extraneous matters, and it was this power of mind that especially appealed to the attorney. Pick out your squirrel and chase him up till you lay hands on him, no matter if Creation falls about your ears while doing it!

CHAPTER XVII

Conclusion

ONE THING TO AVOID – HYPNOTISM A POPULAR
BUGBEAR – WHY IT NEED NOT BE FEARED – NATURAL
HEALING RISES ABOVE LOW PLANE ON WHICH
HYPNOTISM STANDS – TRUE INFLUENCE OVER
FELLOW MEN A NOBLE THING – THE ONENESS WITH
THE INFINITE – FINIS

All schools of medicine as well as all classes of thinkers
are today beginning to recognize suggestion as of the greatest
value not only in physical ailments, but in higher relations of
mind and spirit. There is, however, a widespread fear or distrust
of one feature of suggestion, which is unfortunately one of the
first to present itself to the minds of many people. The word
hypnotism is a great bugbear to many who would otherwise avail
themselves gladly of the help that suggestive therapeutics offers.
Hypnotic suggestions are used by some suggestionists and
practitioners with excellent effect, it is claimed, but in general,
hypnotism is a low plane of suggestion and neither as efficacious
or as safe as the class of suggestive phenomena with which this
work has been dealing. The term hypnotic suggestion is used to
designate a mild hypnosis or state of induced sleep in which the
objective function is lulled to rest and with it the will.

Hypnotic suggestions are extraneous and do not reach
the subjective entity through the will of the patient himself. The
essential quality of hypnotic suggestion is servitude or the
abasement of the individual to the will of another. Pure
suggestion, on the other hand, sets free the will of the patient,
gives him the key to his own power and makes him in the
highest sense master of his own destiny. It arouses the God
within himself, the spirit that is part of the divine whole, instead

of making him subservient to the will of another.

When the soul has been set free by the power of true suggestion it has no need for the lower plane of hypnosis and the greater the spiritual development, the less hold hypnotic suggestion can possibly have upon a person. It cannot be doubted that to the low spiritual development, hypnotic power might offer a real menace, because in the hands of the unscrupulous, the mastery of another's will might offer deep temptation to moral wrong and perversion. But as the soul development rises higher, the danger from hypnotic suggestion or hypnotism in general decreases. No one can be hypnotized against his own will. Hypnosis cannot be induced in anybody without his own acquiescence. Hypnosis predicates concentration upon the part of the person to be hypnotized. When once a person has been hypnotized, and has surrendered his will to the hypnotist, it becomes increasingly easier for the latter to control his subject on future occasions.

But unless one yields and himself consents to the process of concentration which is necessary, he cannot be hypnotized by any one. While in the hands of a perfectly pure and high-minded hypnotist, there might be occasions when hypnotic suggestions would be useful, yet in its basic idea it is a dangerous thing, and especially so to the undeveloped mind. The higher ego, once it is set free by a right understanding and practice of the true suggestion which aims only to make the individual master of himself and not the servant of another, rises above the petty plane of hypnosis into the higher realization of the forces that govern life. What is the need of taking the risks that must appertain to a state whose basic idea is the surrender of volition and servitude to another's will, either for good or bad, when we can be ourselves and reign in our own heritage by the might of our own powers! Everywhere there is advertised instruction in the method of inducing hypnosis, and always the advertisement impresses upon the reader the fact that by this means he can control the actions of others- not that he can do good to humanity, but that he can influence others to his own ends.

The scope and power of hypnotism are always exaggerated and it is made to appear that any one by a short period of study can exercise an unlimited empire over the actions of others regardless of their submission or acquiescence. This is in no sense true, and while hypnotism in unscrupulous hands might work injury to a certain class of subjects, those versed in the higher functions of the subjective entity need have no fear of hypnosis nor desire to use it.

True influence over our fellow men is attained by the force of what we are ourselves, not by submerging the volition of others. Character and personality and not the mysterious balderdash of the platform hypnotist are the real secrets of power among men. These attributes are secured by the development of the divine spirit within ourselves and not by surrender of our birthright to another who may be pure in heart and who may not. In conclusion, I would repeat the premises with which I began this volume: that the Subjective mind rules the functions of the body as well as the emotions and spiritual growth. The Subjective mind is always amenable to Objective suggestions imparted through the medium of the will. The Power which makes us whole physically is the same as that which makes us spiritually ennobled and that Power is within ourselves- it is the Ego, the Spark of the Divine. Whoever will seek, shall find the secret of life in the midst of his own being and by being himself he shall find his amity with the Eternal!

THE END